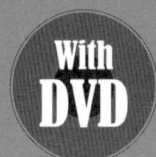

Neurodance-
Exercise for People with Parkinson's Disease

Edited by
Shinichi Takabatake and Hideki Miyaguchi

Choreography
Hiroko Hashimoto

Illustration
Seiko Mesaki

三輪書店
Miwa-Shoten

Miwa-Shoten Ltd.
6-17-9 Hongo Bunkyo-ku, Tokyo
Japan 113-0033

Neurodance-Exercise for People with Parkinson's Disease

Copyright © 2014 by Miwa-Shoten Ltd.
All rights reserved. No part of this publication may be reproduced or transmitted in any form or by any means, electric or mechanical, including photocopying, recording, or any information storage and retrieval system, without permission in writing from the publisher.

ISBN978-4-89590-478-0

This book is based on "Parkinson-Byou ha Kousureba Kawaru (2012)" 〔How to Cope with Symptoms of Parkinson's Disease〕 and translated from Japanese to English.
本書は，高畑進一・宮口英樹（編）『パーキンソン病はこうすれば変わる！―日常生活の工夫とパーキンソンダンスで生活機能を改善』（三輪書店，2012）を再構成し，翻訳したものです．

　The healthcare field is always progressing. Readers are advised to check new theories, therapy and treatment to incorporate these into their own practices. It is the responsibility of the practitioner or therapist, relying on their own experience and knowledge of the patient, to make diagnoses, to determine the best treatment for each individual patient, and to take all appropriate safety precautions. To the fullest extent of the law, neither the publisher nor editor nor author assumes any liability for any injury and/or damage to persons or property arising out of or related to any use of the material contained in this book.
The Publisher

　医学・医療の領域で扱われる知見は，常に変化しています．読者の皆様は，常に新しい理論，療法，治療等を実践に応用していただくため，これらの最新の情報にご注意ください．またご自身の責任のもと，知識・経験にもとづいた実践をされ，安全に対する適切な予防措置を講じてくださるようお願い申し上げます．本書に含まれる内容を運用・実践したことにより，人や財産等に対して何らかの被害・損害が発生した場合でも，出版者，編集者，著者はいかなる責任も負いかねます．　出版者

Contents

Contributors・v
Preface・vi

Part 1 Disability of Daily Movements and Activities in Patients with Parkinson's Disease

Chapter1　Ideas for Daily Movements and Activities in Patients with Parkinson's Disease ·· 2
　Introduction ·· 2
　Common Movements and Activities that are Difficult for Patients with Parkinson's Disease ·· 3
　Ideas for Daily Movements and Activities ·· 7
　Dressing 11/Using the Toilet 13/Bathing 15/Eating 17/Grooming 19/ Getting up, Rising up 21/Walking 1 23/Walking 2 25/Using Public Transportation 27/Doing Housework 1 29/Doing Housework 2 31/ Communicating 33/Enjoying Life 35/Modifying the Home 37/Experiencing Stress and How it Changes Movement 39

Chapter2　Characteristics of Movements and Activities in Patients with Parkinson's Disease ·· 40
　Troubles that Patients Have in Their Daily Lives ·· 40
　Movements and Activities that Patients were used to Become Difficult ·· 40
　Summary ·· 45

Part 2 Understanding Parkinson's Disease

Chapter1　Assessment of Parkinson's Disease: Functional Evaluation of Parkinson's Disease ·· 48
　Severity Rating ·· 48
　Functional Evaluation ·· 49

Chapter2　Assessment of Parkinson's Disease: Assessment of Body Schema Manuscript ·· 55

  Body Schema ·· 55
  Body Schema Assessment Methods ··· 56
  Regarding Body Schema Assessment Methods ······························ 58

Chapter3 Assessment of Parkinson's Disease:
 Evaluation of Motor Imagery ·· 61
  Motor Imagery ·· 61
  Evaluation of Motor Imagery ·· 61
  Motor Imagery of Parkinson's Disease Patients ······························ 62
  Summary ·· 65

Part 3 Neurodance-Exercise for People with Parkinson's Disease

Chapter1 Elements and Structure of the Dance Programs
 for Parkinson's Disease ·· 68
  Introduction ·· 68
  Characteristics of PD and Structure of the Neurodance ················ 68
  Elements Necessary for the PD dance ·· 69
  Structure of the Neurodance ··· 71
  Conclusion ·· 72

Chapter2 The Effectiveness of Dance for the People with
 Parkinson's Disease ··· 74
  Introduction ·· 74
  The Effectiveness of the Neurodance for People with
   Parkinson's Disease ·· 77
  Why the Neurodance is Effective in PD Patients? ························· 81

Chapter3 Video DVD "Let's Enjoy PD Dance!": Description of the
 Contents and Points ·· 84
  1: The Stretch and Relax Dance 85/2: The Patting Dance 86/3: The Heel and Toe Dance 87/4: The Arm and Finger Dance 89/5: The Hand towel Dance 90/6: The Balance Dance 93/7: The Walking Dance 94/8: The Swaying Dance 95

Contributors

Shinichi Takabatake	Osaka Prefecture University
Yasuo Naito	Osaka Prefecture University
Yoshie Tomatsu	Health Welfare Bureau Health Part, Sakai City, Osaka
Tomoko Nishikawa	Osaka Prefecture University
Aiko Hosomoto	Senritsukumodai Homevisit Nursing Station
Hiroyuki Muta	Wakakusa-tatsuma Rehabilitation Hospital
Hiroaki Tanaka	Osaka Prefecture University
Hajime Nakanishi	Hiroshima University Hospital
Fumika Makio	Pref. Osaka Saiseikai Izuo Hospital
Hideki Miyaguchi	Hiroshima University
Hiroko Hashimoto	Aino University

This work was supported in part by Research Grant of Japanese association of occupational therapists (2011-2012) and Grant-in-Aid for Scientific Research (23650325 : 2012-2013), administered by the Ministry of Education, Culture, Sports, Science and Technology, Japan.

Preface

This book describes the difficulties that patients with Parkinson's disease experience in their daily lives, from their assistive devices to the latest therapies and rehabilitations as well as evaluation and intervention methods that focus on body schema and motor imagery and newly developed Neurodance for Parkinson's disease.

This book is filled with thoughts from patients as well as their families and supporters. Part 1 will certainly be helpful for patients, families, and supporters looking for advice about tips and ideas used in daily living. In addition, Part 2 is useful for medical and social welfare professionals who help patients to understand the symptoms and disorders of Parkinson's disease from a novel perspective. Moreover, the concrete methods presented in Part 3 and the attached DVD will certainly help patients and their supporters who are thinking of adopting Neurodance for Parkinson's disease as a training method.

The editors have worked with people with Parkinson's disease for ten years in Osaka and Hiroshima. Ten years ago, Parkinson's disease was considered "a disease with tremor, rigidity, akinesia, and posture adjustment disorder as its main symptoms, which cause difficulty in walking and standing up." However, our patients have taught us that strange and varied phenomena occur in their daily lives. For this reason, the editors, together with occupational therapists, interviewed more than 150 patients and their family members. These interviews revealed various difficulties patients faced in situations other than walking, and showed that patients had developed unique devices to reduce these difficulties. These interviews also revealed characteristics common among patients, such as the importance of motor imagery and visual information, weak attention distribution, vulnerability of body schema, and susceptible mentality and emotions. Surprisingly, these factors were the very topics whose mechanisms have been elucidated in recent neuroscience advances.

Therefore, we wondered if it would be possible to adopt those factors receiving attention in neuroscience research to dance. We first investigated which dance characteristics were most effective against Parkinson's disease. Because there are various kinds of dance, we needed to analyze dance movements and methods to devise the most effective dance for patients. In the course of our investigation, hints were found in the phenomena that occur in patients and their devices, particularly the idea of utilizing body schema and motor imagery. Our investigation identified dance factors to counter problems that arise due to the interaction disorder between basal ganglia and the frontal lobe, under the hypothesis that "dance enhances body schema and motor imagery of patients, and facilitates their planning and practice of exercises." We developed Neurodance based these ideas and perfected it through repeated trials and modifications in cooperation with the Patients Association.

We believe that dancing improves patient body schema and motor imagery and influences mental and physical functions. Chapter 2 of Part 3 describes our examination of these effects in cooperation with the Patients Association.

Lastly, we would like to express our sincere gratitude to the patients and families who cooperated with and contributed to the production of this book and DVD. We also thank the specialists whose discussions provided us with increased awareness and new ideas.

May 2014, Editor

Part 1

Disability of Daily Movements and Activities in Patients with Parkinson's Disease

1 Ideas for Daily Movements and Activities in Patients with Parkinson's Disease

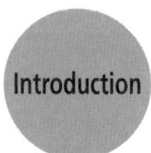
Introduction

What is Parkinson's Disease (PD) ?

PD is a degenerative disorder of the central nervous system. The motor symptoms of PD result from a lack of dopamine. PD is more common in the elderly, with most cases occurring between the ages of 50-60.

Common symptoms are movement-related: these include shaking, muscle rigidity, slow movements, and impaired posture and balance.

Treatment of PD

There are medications which can relieve the symptoms in addition to multidisciplinary management. After consulting a doctor, proper medication will effectively manage symptoms.

It is best to continue various activities in daily life. Doing this will improve the symptoms or keep them from becoming worse. Try to take care of yourself as much as possible.

Continue to move your body: exercising, dancing and walking are effective ways to maintain and improve your movements.

For Those Reading This Book

We asked patients with PD, "What movements or activities do you feel are difficult in your daily life?" and "What makes those movements or activities easier for you?"

We analyzed their answers and made this book to show the common characteristics for difficult daily movements or activities. There are tips to deal with these movements and activities in a Question-and-Answer format.

This information may not apply to everybody but we hope it will be useful for some people.

Common Movements and Activities that are Difficult for Patients with Parkinson's Disease

1) Movements or activities that are carried out unconsciously are difficult.

If patients with PD are not conscious of their movements or postures, they cannot walk well or keep good posture. For example, when they use chopsticks or scissors, if they are not thinking of the correct way to hold them and move them, they cannot use them well.

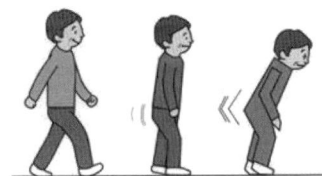

2) Activities with multiple steps are difficult.

At a cash register, we take out money from our wallet and give it to the clerk. Then we receive the change and a receipt and put them in our wallet. Such activities requiring a sequence of steps like this one become difficult to smoothly carry out.

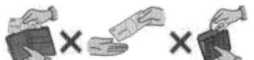

3) Movements or activities that require doing two tasks at the same time are difficult.

Examples are grilling a fish while cutting food, or stepping forward while opening a door.

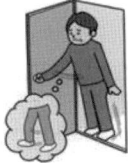

4) Movements and activities that are carried out using both hands are difficult.

Washing your face, putting a letter in an envelope, folding the laundry are examples.

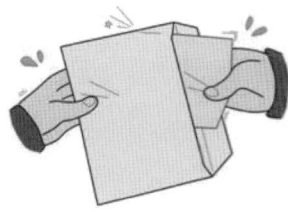

5) Alternating repetitive movements or activities are difficult.

These include brushing your teeth and rubbing your
back with a towel.

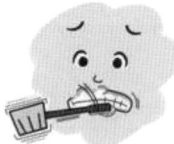

6) Movements or activities repeating the same motion are difficult.

Drawing circles or writing words are examples.
Your handwriting gradually becomes smaller and
smaller.

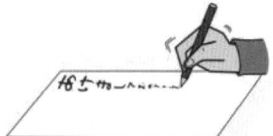

7) Movements or activities that are done without looking at your own body and limbs are difficult.

Raising pants behind a body, rolling over in bed,
walking in a dark place: these movements become
difficult.

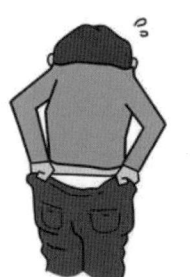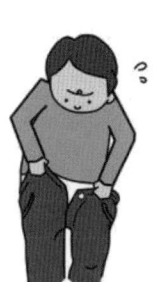

8) Movements or activities without target objects are difficult.

Standing up, walking, rolling over, elevating an arm:
these intransitive movements become difficult.

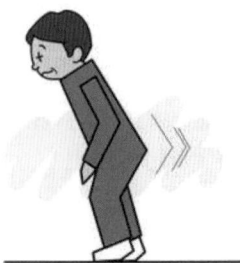

9) Movements or activities toward oneself are difficult.

Lifting up food to the mouth, brushing teeth, shaving, putting on make-up, washing the face, and putting on clothes: these movements become difficult.

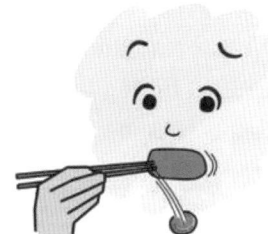

Patients' movements and activities are strongly influenced by surroundings and circumstances.

10) Movements or activities without enough visual information are difficult.

Trying to do something in a dim location or cluttered space: these movements become difficult.

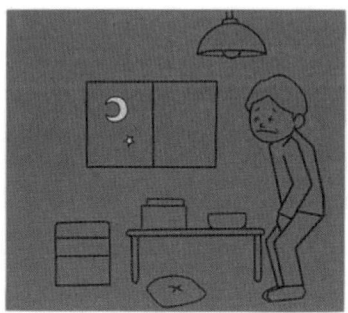

11) Movements or activities are difficult when surroundings change and when the shape of an object changes.

Walking into a narrow corridor from a spacious room; moving in a place where people are walking in various directions; putting objects into a shapeless, soft shopping bag: a change in the sight information is in all these examples.

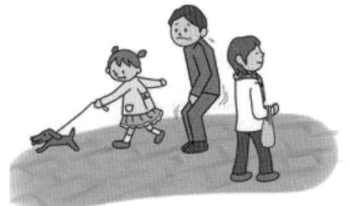

12) Movements or activities to be completed in a place the patient has never been before or in an unusual situation are difficult.

In a restroom away from home, patients cannot sit on the seat just as well as they would do in their own home. If the location of an object is changed, even in their own house, they cannot move well.

13) Movements or activities that require estimating the distance of articles to the patient's body are difficult.

Reaching for a handrail, opening the refrigerator door without hitting themselves with the door: these movements become difficult.

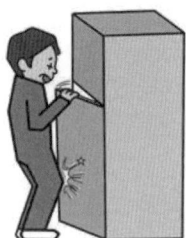

Their movements and activities are strongly influenced by emotions and their psychological condition.

14) Movements or activities under anxiety or with unpleasant feelings are difficult.

When patients hear harsh words or feel uncomfortable, their movements may become impaired.

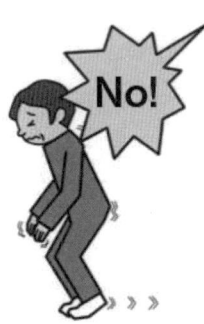

Ideas for Daily Movements and Activities

If you have PD and feel some difficulties in daily life, these ideas may help you. Continue daily life by using various ideas. This is important for rehabilitation.

1) Consciously think about how to move your body, limbs and the tools you are holding.

When you walk, think about how to move your feet and waist. When you use chopsticks or a pencil, be aware of how to hold and move them.

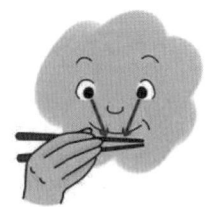

2) Plan procedures and movements before doing them.

Imagine procedures and the needed movements before you actually doing them as follows. 'First, I go to the door. Next, I open the door and then get my luggage' or 'I take out a pen from the drawer. Then I sign the receipt.'

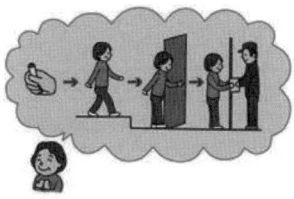

3) Avoid doing multiple movements at the same time.

When you cook, complete one task at a time. First, only boil your vegetables. Next, only fry the fish. At last, grill the meat. It is important that you take enough time to complete each task. Be patient.

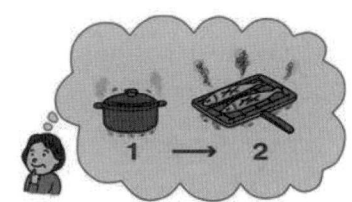

4) Use just one hand if you have difficulty using both hands.

If you have difficulty washing your face or hair with both hands, then simply do it with one hand.

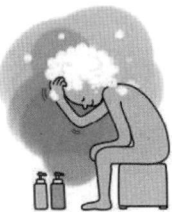

5) Focus on one direction when you do an alternating repetitive movement or activity.

If you have difficulty moving your toothbrush up and down, brush your teeth with a one-way movement from the top to the bottom or from the bottom to the top.

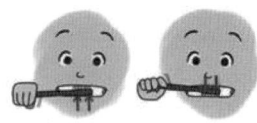

6) When you are repeating the same movement, after some time change or shift the angle of the movement.

If your steps become smaller while you walk, then move your feet in a slightly different direction. You will be able to step smoothly again. Keep your mood positive and do this again and again as you walk.

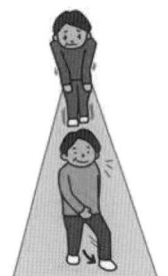

7) When you move, watch your hands, feet and body.

Use a mirror to see how your limbs and body are moving. When you have to move your limbs and body without looking at them, imagine putting strength into your limbs and body first before you move. This will help you confirm that your limbs and body are in position and ready for action.

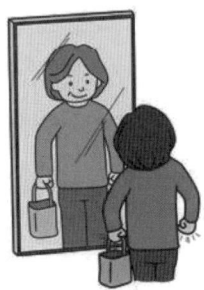

8) Use marks and objects for your movement or activity.

Mark a line on the floor next to your bed. Step over the line on the floor and begin to walk. When you reach your chair, then begin turning your body and sitting down. Stand up while watching your clock on the wall.

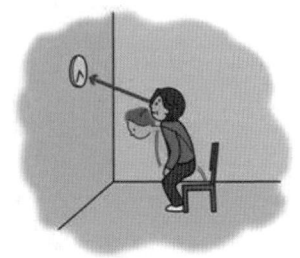

9) When a movement or activity you do by yourself is difficult, do it after touching your face and body.

Touch your face before shaving or putting on makeup. Then imagine your face and yourself doing the task.

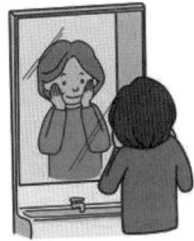

> Know the importance of adjusting your environment to suit your needs.

10) Make sure you can easily see your body, objects and the places you have marked.

Keep your room neat and tidy so it will be easy to see the marks and objects. Turn on the light in the room at night so it will be easy to see them and also your body. Keep bright lights in the room.

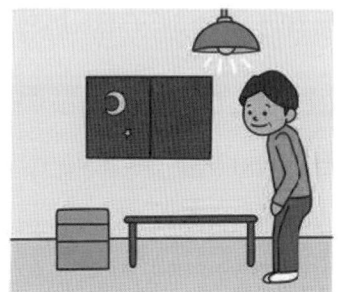

11) Avoid crowded places.

Go out during the time when a train or a shop is not crowded. It is best to use a basket type bag for shopping rather than soft plastic or cloth bag.

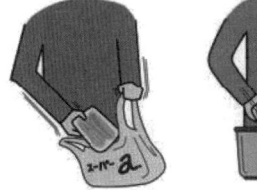

12) Perform regular movements in a familiar environment.

When you clean and tidy up your rooms, it is best to always keep familiar marks and objects in the same place. You will easily be able to do your usual movements and activities.

    Any household repairs or renovation should be done as soon as possible. Then you will be able to get used to the new situation as soon as possible.

    When you move to an unfamiliar place or situation, think about what you want to do first, imagine yourself successfully doing the movements and then do them.

13) Before you move, look at your hands, arms, feet, legs, body, face and objects, and touch them to feel their distances from you.

When you walk between desks or chairs, sit down on a bed or a toilet seat, slightly touch the objects around you.

It is important to enjoy life and stay positive.

14) Positive attitude and good feelings will keep your movements smooth.

Do your favorite sports, hobbies and exciting jobs.

Repeating movements daily will allow you to maintain and improve your movements.

15) You will be able to retain movements by repeating them everyday.

Continue doing your movements and activities everyday. When a movement becomes difficult, you may be able to do it again if you intensively repeat the movement. Some people have been able to knit sweaters again or play a musical instrument again by gradually repeating and carefully practicing the movements everyday.

Column

The movements and activities that patients with PD have difficulty with vary. We analyzed many cases and found 14 kinds of common characteristics and 15 kinds of tasks. Why do these difficulties occur in their everyday lives? We must consider a motor function and a cognitive function of PD when we think about this. The reasons that these difficulties occur and a possible interpretation concerning brain function and how it affects motor and cognitive function are discussed in Part 1, Chapter 2.

Dressing

From the early stages of PD, dressing and undressing are activities that are difficult. Think about your hand movements and how to hold your clothes. Consider the size of your clothes and the kind of fabric they are made from.

Q1. My movement stops when I cannot see my hands and feet.

It is difficult to put on/take off my trousers and to check the back of my skirt or my coat. Movements get difficult when I cannot see my hands inside my clothes. When my foot gets caught on the hem of my pants it is hard to get my foot through and start moving again.

A1. Closely look at or touch your body, arms, and legs.
Use a mirror. Tuck in and bundle your pants or skirt into a "ring" before putting your feet and legs through. You will be able to see your body better and this will allow you to move easier.

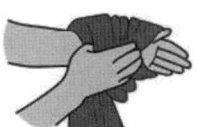
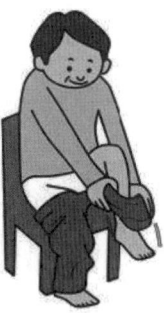

Q2. I cannot put on clothes well when I'm not thinking about what I'm doing.

A2. Decide your movements before you begin, and do them after you imagine yourself doing them.
If you always do the same movements, it will be easy to imagine them.

Q3. It is hard to put on clothes that are rumpled.

A3. Put on clothes only after you have straightened the hem of the pants and the sleeves of a jacket.

Q 4. It takes a lot of time to take off clothes from the top part of my body.

A 4. When you take off a garment over your head, raise it from the "back collar", behind your neck.
When you take off a garment from the sleeves, pull it from the shoulder, not from the cuffs. Choose clothes made of silky fabric that is easy to slip on and off.

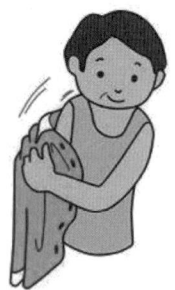

Q 5. I cannot put a button through the buttonhole.

Particularly, it is hard to button the buttons near my neck.

A 5. First confirm the shape of the button and the hole.
Do this by using a mirror or before putting it on or by looking at buttons and buttonholes lower down on your blouse or shirt. As you put the button through the buttonhole, be aware of the movements of both your hands.

Q 6. It takes time to put on socks.

Tuck in and bundle your socks into a "ring" and then put them on as you cover your feet.
Be seated when you put on your socks. Use a low stand to rest your foot upon. Move your foot back and forth from heel to toe as you pull up on the sock.

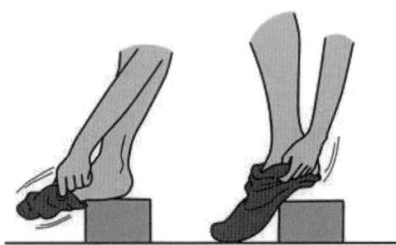

Using the Toilet

In the bathroom, you must do many movements in a small place. Try to keep the area as spacious as possible. Practice your movements.

Q 1. It is difficult to put on/take off my trousers.

Trousers often get stuck at my hips.

A 1. Put your hands inside the trousers and pull them up from behind.
Choose trousers made with stretchy fabric and elastic waistbands without zippers. Wear suspenders and use them to help lift your trousers.

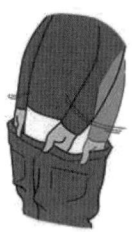

Q 2. I cannot position myself well on toilet seat.

Turning smoothly is impossible in a restroom. The position of my behind often does not match the toilet seat.

A 2. Mark the floor with footprints, for example, to show where your feet should be at each step.
Stand on the footprints and turn around. Stand on the footprints before sitting down. When you change direction, first extend your hand or turn your face, then change the direction of your body. Make sure your calves hit the toilet seat before sitting down.

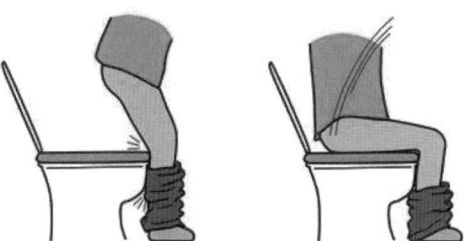

Q 3. It is hard to stand up from toilet seat.

A 3. Imagine standing up before doing it: 'First I have to extend one foot from my body, next bend my body forward, then stand up while extending my body upward.'

Chapter 1   Ideas for Daily Movements and Activities in Patients with Parkinson's Disease

Q4. When I urinate in a standing position, I bend forward.

A4. Make a mark at your eye-level, look at it and imagine yourself with a straight posture.

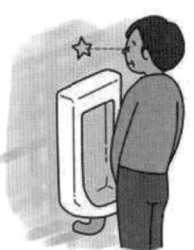

Q5. I cannot smoothly go into and come out of the restroom.

When I open and close the door, I hit my body and almost fall down. I cannot step forward while opening a door.

A5. Put a mark to indicate the position where you should stand when you open or close the door.
Put one hand on a handrail or the wall to help support your body, then open or close the door. Practice performing the movements, one by one.

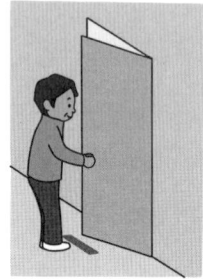

Q6. It is hard to perform movements in a restroom I've never been to before.

A6. Choose a stall that is installed with handrails and is wide.

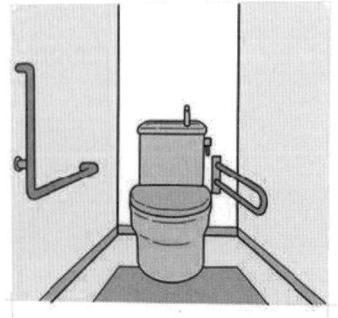

Q7. At night, it is hard to know what direction my restroom is in at home.

A7. Keep the lights on in the hallway and the restroom at night.

Bathing

People take baths in a slippery place. Keep your movements familiar and safe.

Q 1. It is hard to squeeze out the towel.

A 1. Extend your elbows as far as you can while grasping the towel with both hands.

Q 2. It is hard to wash my hair with both hands.

A 2. Wash your hair with one hand while being conscious of your hand's large and slow movement.

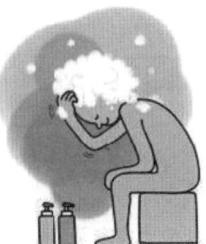

Q 3. I am afraid of closing my eyes. So I cannot shower.

A 3. Shower while sitting on a shower chair with backrest. If you maintain good posture, you will have confidence.
Using a shampoo hat may also help.

Q 4. When I rub my back with a towel, the movement of my hand becomes smaller.

A 4. Hold your towel in both hands, but only move your towel with one hand.

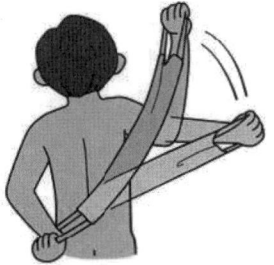

Q 5. When I wipe my body with my towel, I cannot feel any strength going to my hand.

A 5. Wipe your body while you use a mirror to confirm the position of your hand and towel.

Q6. It is hard getting into and out of the bathtub.

A6. First decide on the steps to do to get into and out of your bathtub. Visualize your movements before you carry them out.

Q7. When I feel danger or feel a place is too narrow, my feet freeze up.

A7. Use handrails or anti-slip mats. Keep everything organized and uncluttered in your dressing room and bathroom.
This will help you feel secure.

Q8. If the bathroom is slightly dark, my movement stops.

A8. Keep the area bright.

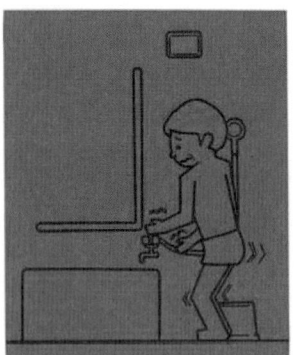 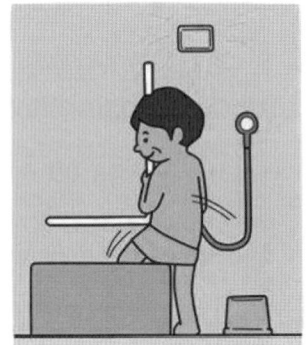

Eating

Using chopsticks or a spoon requires control. Try to maintain good posture while eating.

Q 1. I can lift food near my mouth, but I spill it when I lose sight of it around my lips.

A 1. Try using a mirror to see your mouth.

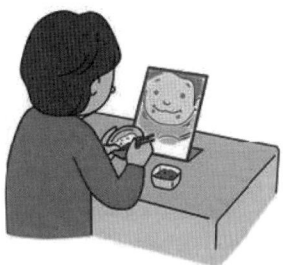

Q 2. I have a bad sense of distance. My chopsticks and spoon hit the edge of my mouth.

A 2. Look at the tip of chopsticks or the tip of the spoon. Move your hand while you confirm the distance.

Q 3. My hand stops when I repeat the movement to lift food to my mouth. Gradually, my mouth becomes hard to open.

A 3. Put down your chopsticks and raise your hands high. Then start eating again. Massage your face before start eating.

Q 4. When eating, my chopsticks trouble me.

A 4. Hold one chopstick and move it as you use a pencil. Stop your hand and re-grip correctly. When your chopsticks are parallel, you cannot move them effectively. Please confirm how to grasp them so that the tips of chopsticks meet.

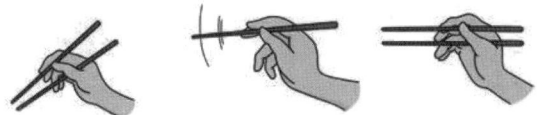

Q5. My body gradually inclines during a meal.

A5. Consciously correct your posture. Focus on any vertical lines on a piece of furniture or an appliance to adjust your posture from time to time.

Chairs with armrests help, too.

Grooming

Keep yourself neat to enjoy your everyday life and stay active. Be conscious of your hand movements and how you hold your grooming supplies.

Q1. When I wash my face, I feel like I don't have enough strength.

A1. Use one hand if using both hands seems difficult.
Wash your face after first touching your face with your hands, as you were checking the shape of your face.

Q2. I almost fall down if I close my eyes when I wash my face.

A2. Hold the edge of the sink or handrail with one hand. Wash your face with the other hand.

Q3. When I brush my teeth I cannot maintain rhythm.

A3. Focus on one direction, for instance just up or just down.
Pay attention not only to your hands, but also to how you are adjusting the position of your neck.

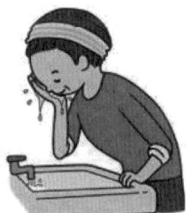

Q4. It is difficult for me to adjust the angle of my shaver to my face and my toothbrush to my teeth.

A4. Use a mirror to confirm the direction you are holding your shaver or toothbrush.
Shave your beard or brush your teeth after touching your face with your hands, as if you were checking the shape of your face.

Q5. My hand freezes up when I brush my teeth and wash my face while I am standing.

A5. Place a chair in the room. Brush your teeth and wash your face while you sit.

Q 6. When I put on my makeup, I feel that even a sponge is heavy.

  A 6. Use a cotton ball. Apply your makeup with one hand.

Q 7. When I'm feeling down, it's hard to put on my makeup.

  A 7. If you are motivated, it will ease your movement.
  Having many opportunities to happily interact with people is important for you to feel better.

Getting up, Rising up

Walking, getting up and rising up are frequent everyday movements and are also required for bathing and using the toilet. Be conscious of your body movement. Learn how to deal with your bedding.

Q 1. I cannot smoothly roll over and rise up.

A 1. Do it while consciously thinking about how to move your body, limbs and head.
Touch the bed with your hand while you think about the sequence of positions. First imagine what you will do. 1) Turn down blanket, 2) twist your upper body to get in a lateral posture, 3) bring down both legs from the bed, and 4) extend an elbow and push up the upper body. Choose a moderately hard mattress. An electric bed that elevates your head is useful.

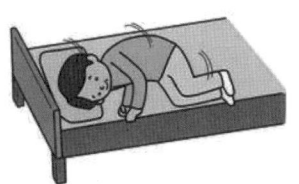 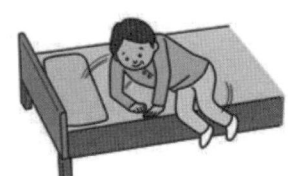 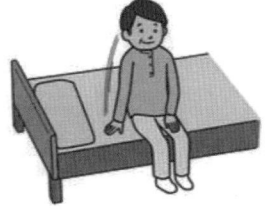

Q 2. Especially at night, I feel it is difficult to sit up, rise up and walk.

A 2. Even at night, keep a light on in the room so you can see the furniture and door.

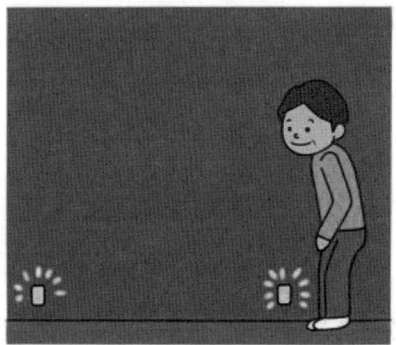

Q 3. My blanket seems to cling to my body, and getting up is hard for me. I feel that even a light blanket is very heavy.

A 3. Use light blankets that do not cling to you.
Use sheets and blankets made of silky smooth material.

Q 4. When my body is covered with a blanket I cannot move, because I cannot see where my hands and feet are.

A 4. Before you move under the blanket, think about putting strength into you limbs and body and tightening your muscles.
Before you start getting up, first take out your fingers and toes from under the blanket.

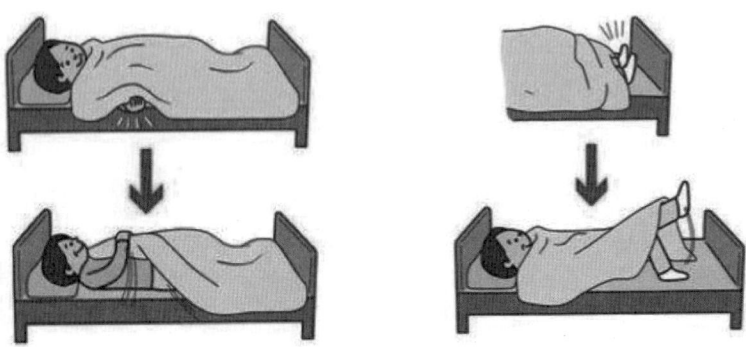

Q 5. After I have sat for a long time, it is hard to stand up.

A 5. Stand up while thinking about rounding your body and bending it forward.
It becomes easy to stand up when you look at a mark on the floor and wall.

Walking 1

Walking is a fundamental activity. Make sure you feel comfortable when you walk. Make changes in your environment.

Q 1. I freeze up when I begin to walk.

A 1. Say some words to encourage yourself before you take a step. As you walk match your feet to the lines on the floor.
Before you start walking, first take one step backwards and then take a step diagonally.

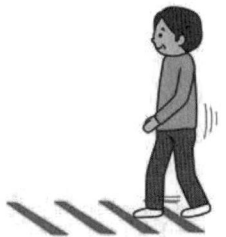 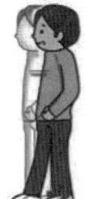

Q 2. I freeze up in front of a step or a narrow passage.

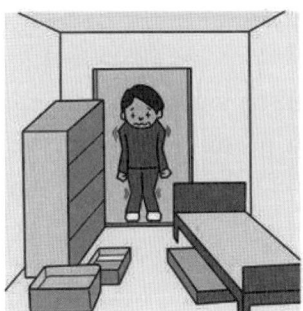

A 2. Before you walk, imagine how to move your limbs and body.
Before walking, try guessing how many steps you will need to take to arrive at the door. Try imagining the movements when you step over the steps, then perform it. Rearrange and tidy up your rooms to make them as spacious as possible.

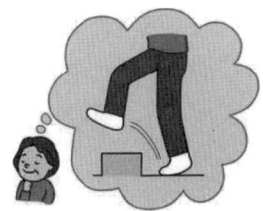

Q 3. When I move into a narrow place from a wide place, I freeze up.

A 3. Stop once, and confirm the width of the narrow space.
Look and also touch the edges of the door.

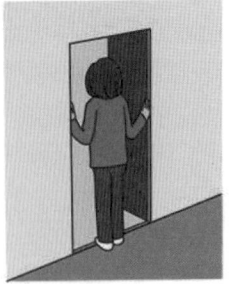

Q 4. I have difficulty changing directions when I walk.

A 4. Face the direction you wish to go in before pivoting your body.
Use a mark to move your eyes and turn your face.

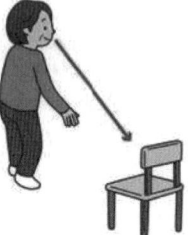

Q 5. It becomes hard to walk when I am not conscious of my movements.

A 5. Be conscious of your joint and muscular movements and also the balance of your body.
Lift up one thigh and be aware of putting down your foot from your heel first. Straighten your posture and be aware of walking by slowly striding along.

Walking 2

Q 6. It becomes hard to walk when I carry something.

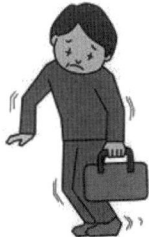

A 6. When you are carrying an item, try to find the position you can balance your body.
Use a shoulder bag or a backpack instead of carrying a bag on your forearm.

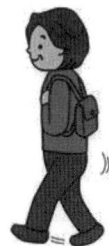

Q 7. It is hard to walk on a sidewalk, which gently curves.

A 7. Try to think about the difference between stepping with your right foot and then stepping with your left foot.
Step forward as you use the lines in the sidewalk surface as a mark.

Q 8. I cannot walk very well in crowded places.

A 8. Do not pay too much attention to people walking around you. Instead, pay attention to where you are going.

Q 9. I cannot walk well when I am in a hurry and when I get impatient.

A 9. Be aware of how to move your body as discussed in **Walking 1**.
Then take a deep breath, relax and think "Let's walk."

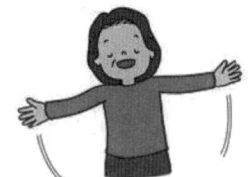

Q 10. I freeze up when I only think, "It is slippery and seems dangerous."

A 10. Try to make things easier and safe.
Attach a safeguard and a handrail. Make all your rooms well lit. Place the furniture in a way so that you can see everything. Carry a walking stick for your safety. When you go outdoors, choose wide and safe paths.

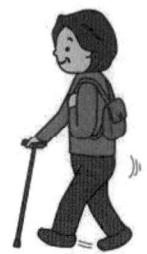

Q 11. I cannot move well even if I have a helper assist me.

A 11. It is effective if the helper helps you by using a visual mark and by concrete words to encourage your motor imagery.
It is better if your helper tells you specifically to lift up your right/left thigh while you are imagining that, instead of only telling you to walk. It is important that your helper shows you the place where to put your hand and your foot. Your helper should use marks and point to them.

Using Public Transportation

Public transportation is an essential part of our lives. Cars and bicycles are also important. Use them safely after carefully devising a procedure and practicing the movements.

Train and Bus

Q 1. I cannot smoothly get off the train.

A 1. Before the train arrives at the station, prepare yourself to get off the train.
Note which doors will open, move close to the doors and face towards the doors.

Q 2. It is hard to pass through a narrow automatic ticket gate at a station.

A 2. Go through the ticket gate after you imagine your movements doing it. Touch the automatic ticket gate with your hands as you walk through.

Q 3. When I buy a ticket, I have trouble taking my money out of my wallet.

A 3. Use a prepaid card.

Driving a Car

Q 4. While I drive I can see the centerline and the white line along the sidewalk, but I cannot drive my car straight. My car veers to one side. Because I cannot accurately perceive depth and width, I cannot skillfully drive in reverse. I cannot drive well in unfamiliar surroundings.

A 4. See, below.

Driving a Motorcycle and Riding a Bicycle

Q 5. I am good at riding a bicycle, but when I have to ride through a narrow way or small area, it becomes difficult.

I do not know how to pass by a car or a person. When a person or a car suddenly appears, I freeze up and cannot deal with the situation.

A4·A5. Being able to get around independently is important, but more important is everyone's safety.

First judge if driving a car, motorcycle or riding a bicycle is safe for everyone.

Doing Housework 1

Housework consists of complicated procedures. Therefore PD often affects it in the early stage of the disease. Get useful tools and arrange your surroundings. Slowly and carefully think about the steps of housework before you do them.

Cooking

Q1. It is difficult to do two activities simultaneously, for example, grilling fish while cooking another dish.

A1. Imagine the cooking procedures beforehand.
Write down the steps. Rehearse them in your mind before you start cooking your dishes. For each step, first take out the things you need, such as utensils, ingredients and seasoning. It is very important to focus on each step. Use your cookbooks to check your steps while you are cooking. Use books with pictures of utensils and ingredients, books with illustrations for each step and electronic devices that show the ingredients and the procedures.

Q2. It is not possible to mix an egg well.

A2. Be conscious about what you are doing when you move your chopsticks in one direction.

Doing the Laundry

Q3. I cannot hang the laundry on hangers.

A3. Put and flatten one piece of laundry on a table or desk, then put a hanger through it.

Q 4. When I fold clothes, I end up messing them all up.

It is difficult to put corners together. I cannot remember the procedure to put the clothes down.

A 4. Check the folding steps first.

Hold down the clothes on a table with one hand and match the corners with the other. Use illustrations or tools that help with folding. One idea is to use tools such as the clothes folding board or Quick Press.

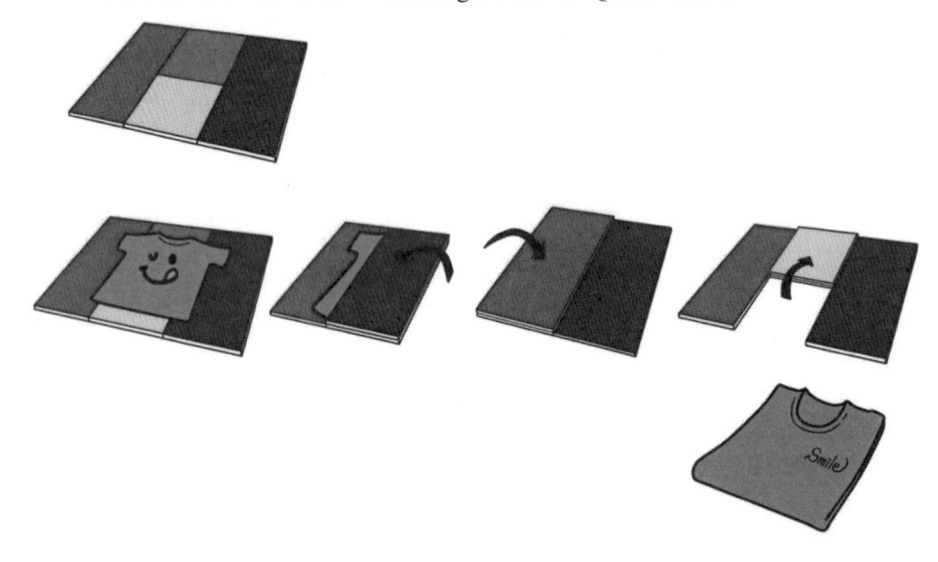

Doing Housework 2

Shopping

Paying Money

Q 5. I cannot smoothly take my wallet out of my bag.

  A 5. When you put your wallet into your bag, always put it in the same place or pocket.

Q 6. It is hard to take out some coins and bills from my wallet at a cash register. I get upset.

My hand does not move at all when I get upset.

  A 6. When you pay, prepare it beforehand.
  Be conscious of which procedure you will do first, taking out coins or taking out bills. Perform just one task at a time. Put coins on your palm and let the cashier take the coins from your hand. You can also use electronic money to pay.

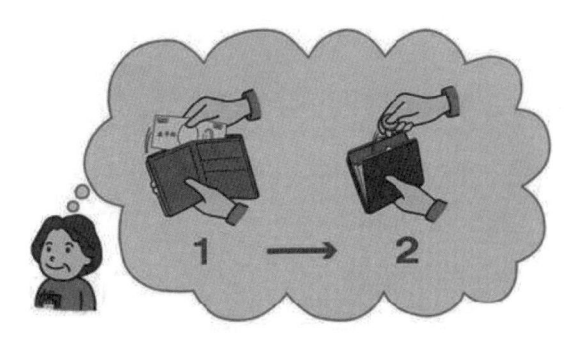

Putting Things in a Shopping Bag

Q 7. When I am putting groceries into a bag, I have a hard time keeping the bag open.

I also get confused about which items should go in what order and how.

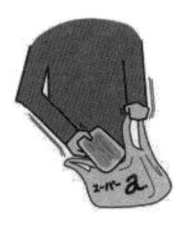

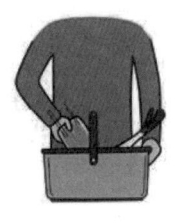

  A 7. Bring your own bag that is basket-shaped so you can see your hand movements as well as the shape of the items. See-through baskets are recommended.

Clear, non-flexible bags with a solid form are recommended.

Cleaning up

Q 8. I cannot clean up a room as skillfully as I used to do. I do not know why, but it takes many hours. Though I intend to clean it well, the room is not cleaned up at all.

A 8. Decide a place for each object to be.

Keep each object in the same place. After your room is as you like it, take a photograph of it to help you remember.

Responding to Visitors

Q 9. When the doorbell rings, I try to answer it right away but cannot figure out what to do. Then I freeze up.

A 9. Ahead of time, ask your visitor to let you know when he/she will be coming over.

Before your visitor arrives, go through the steps in your head.

For example, when a package is being delivered: "Get my pen, go to the entrance, open the door, sign the receipt, receive the package and close the door."

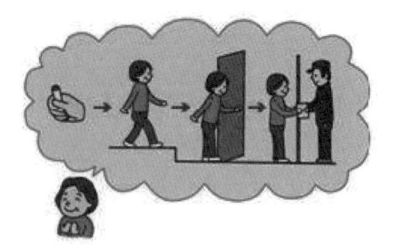

Communicating

Writing, using a computer, and speaking are all important methods of communication. Consciously think about how to move your fingers, mouth and tools.

Q 1. It has become hard to hit the keys on the keyboard of my PC with both hands.

  A 1. Switch to a method using one hand.
  Change the keyboard setting for one hand input.

Q 2. I cannot use a computer mouse well.

  A 2. Change the keyboard setting. Mouse operation can be done with a numeric keypad.
  Using a PC that you can operate with a touch panel is one idea.

Q 3. When I write on blank paper, the letters are distorted. But when I do calligraphy, my hobby, I can do it with no problem.

  A 3. Like doing calligraphy, picture where and how you will be writing before you start.
  Be conscious of what you are doing, write your letters in the center of a ruled line and write big. Still if it is difficult, change the ruled line to a color that is easy to notice.

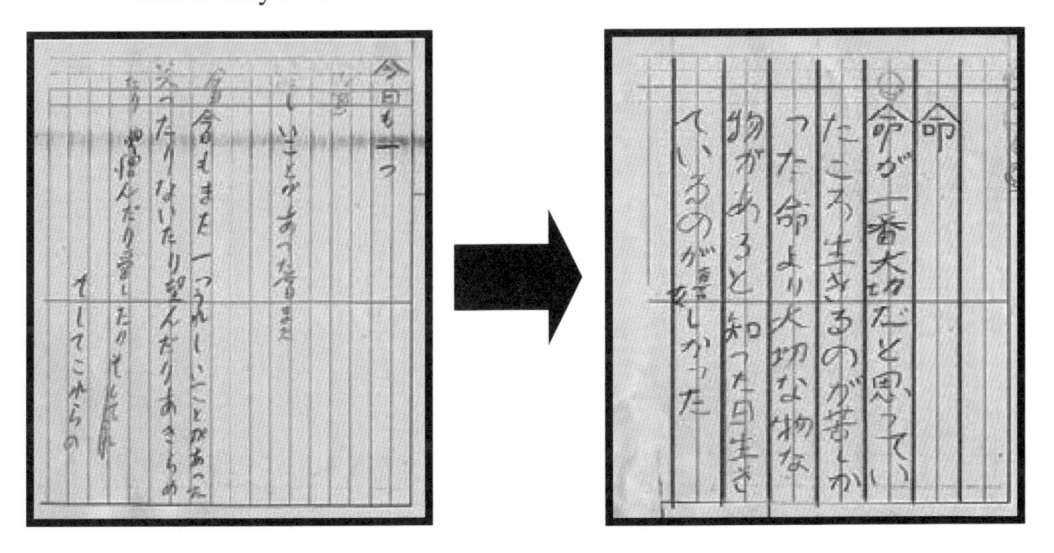

Q4. When I write with a pen, the strength in my hand is too great and the characters gradually become small.

A4. Write being conscious of how you hold your pen, how much strength you are putting into your grip and the size of your letters.

Q5. I cannot write many words at one time.

A5. First, put your pen down and relax your hand.
Then hold your pen again. Write slowly while you think about when to add strength to your grip and when to relax. Be conscious of how your fingers hold your pen and how your hand moves across the paper.

Q6. I cannot put a letter in an envelope well. I do not know why, but the letter hits the edge of the envelope. I cannot smoothly put documents in a clear file either.

A6. Put the envelope on a desk. Hold the envelope in one place with one hand.
Match the letter with the edge of the envelope with your other hand. Do the same with a Plastic folder.

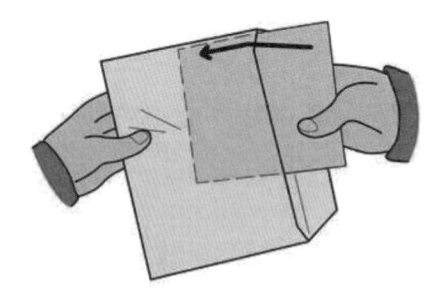

Q7. It is hard for me to speak because my lips do not move smoothly.

A7. Be aware of your lips and their movement as you talk.
Singing in a loud voice will improve lip movement.

Enjoying Life

Your work and hobbies are important. They give you strength.

Q 1. Is it better to quit my work or hobby so that my disease does not worsen?

A 1. Repeating your movements helps you maintain and improve your movements. Continue with your everyday life and favorite activities because the actions you repeat everyday will stay with you longer than those you do not repeat. Stay active.
［Comments from patients with PD］
 a. When I worked, I did not feel symptoms of PD frequently, so my colleagues did not notice that I was sick. However, the opportunities to go out decreased after I quit work, and the disease suddenly progressed.
 b. Because I dance and do kendo, I don't have any problems with my posture.
 c. My voice has become stronger since I began to sing karaoke. I can better control the saliva spilling from my mouth, too.

Q 2. Usually I cannot move very well, but I can move really well when I am concentrating on my favorite hobby. This difference is extreme. Therefore, some neighbors misunderstand me. They think I am lazy or selfish.

A 2. Feelings and psychological conditions strongly influence the movements of patients with PD. Therefore, a difference can be seen in the movements and this sometimes causes other people's misunderstandings. Continue working in the garden, participating in sports, dancing, and doing your favorite hobby including karaoke. It is important to continue doing worthwhile work and be with reliable friends.
［Comments from patients with PD］
 a. I love trips. When traveling, I feel I'm in good condition and can walk more smoothly than usual. My family is surprised at this difference.
 b. When I go fishing, I can walk while I carry heavy baggage.
 c. Though it is difficult to walk in my home, I can run after a ball quickly and can hit the ball when I play table tennis. I feel this is very strange.
 d. When I put on new clothes and accessories, I feel happy and excited. My feet become light and I can move them easier.

e. When I am with my favorite people, I can easily move my body.

f. If I have a goal like the target in mini-golf, or if I am competing to win in sports, it is easy for me to move my body.

Modifying the Home

Take advantage of home modification and welfare equipment that can help your everyday movements.

Q 1. Is it effective to have handrails installed and use welfare equipment?

A 1. To ensure safety, have handrails installed and start using welfare equipment.
You will get a sense of safety and will avoid awkward movements. In addition, handrails can support you as well as be a mark for your movements.

Q 2. When should I start modifying my home and using welfare equipment?

A 2. Start as early as possible, to get used to the modifications and the equipment.
Install a toilet seat with a cleaning function and handrails in your restroom. Use welfare equipment such as a walking stick or nursing bed from an early stage.

Q 3. What should I be careful of when taking advantage of home modification and welfare equipment?

A 3. It is important for patients with PD to do the same behavior as much as possible in a familiar environment. Use equipment to support your regular movements.
Have handrails installed at places where you usually put your hands. Installing too many handrails may disturb your movement. Put a chair in the bathroom, if it will help your movement.

Q 4. Is there anything else to do?

A 4. Arrange and tidy up your room and keep the areas you move around in clear and spacious. Furniture and other articles that you use as marks are always essential for your movement. When you ask somebody to arrange them, you should confirm where to place them.

Keep your bed and chair in the same place so you will be able to repeat the same usual movements. Install a mark on the floor or wall indicating the places to put your feet and the places to pay careful attention.

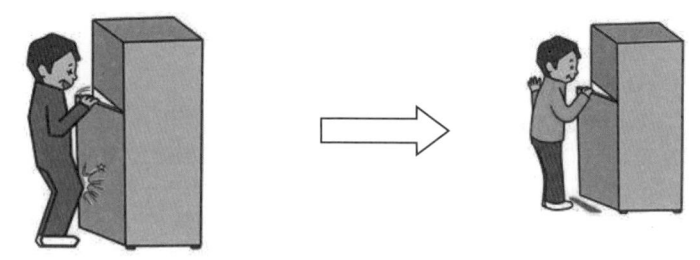

Keep lights in the rooms and hallways on at night. Install large mirrors so you can see your limb movements and your posture.

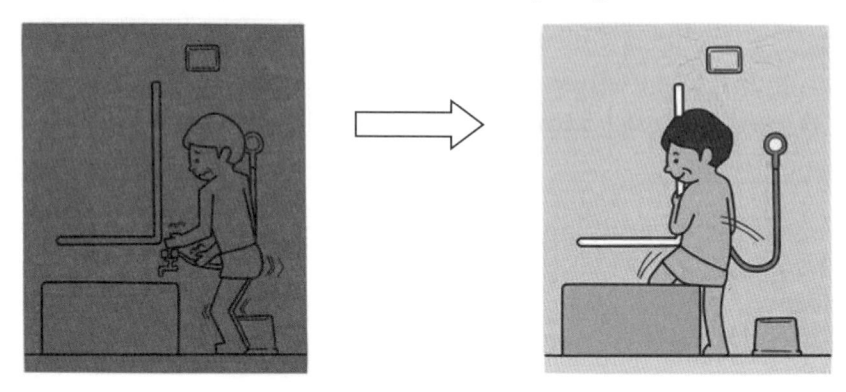

Patients often lose balance when a road surface or floor inclines. Stairs are easier and safer to use.

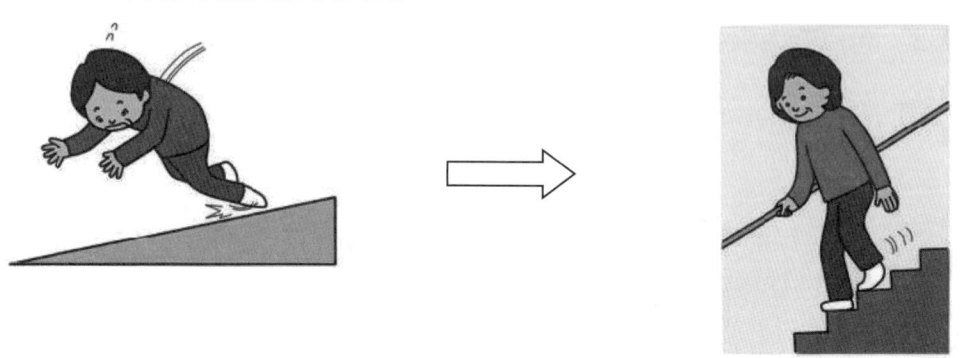

Experiencing Stress and How it Changes Movement

For patients, moderate feelings of strain may help make movements smooth, but excessive tension or stress disturbs movement. Keep in mind to stay relaxed and to keep moving.

Q 1. I cannot move when I'm in a hurry and when someone says something unpleasant.

I only think about the unpleasant thing that was said, and it becomes hard for me to move. I cannot move when I am tense.

A 1. Do deep breathing and calm your heart. Keep in mind to move slowly. Do work or housework when you are feeling well. Tell your family and helper that nervous tension disturbs your movements and optimism enables you to move better.

Q 2. What can the family and helper do for the patient with PD?

A 2. "He could do it a little while ago. Why is he unable to do it now?" "She can move in front of the doctor. Why not in front of me?" "Is he lazy?" We often hear these comments from families of patients with PD. Their ability to move changes greatly depending on time and place. Most families are confused and puzzled by this. This is characteristic of patients who have PD. It is important to watch the movements of your family member with PD. Listen to them when a movement is difficult and when they tell you how it becomes easier to move if you support them.

"Hurry up, hurry up." When you rush patients with PD, they may become nervous and it will be more difficult for them to move. Their movements strongly depend on their mood and feelings. Sometimes it is important to respect the pace of the patient.

Also, promote movement by saying concrete words. Instead of saying "Come on, walk," it is better to say "Raise your right thigh." It is effective to use specific words.

(Shinichi Takabatake, Yasuo Naito, Yoshie Tomatsu, Tomoko Nishikawa, Aiko Hosomoto, Hiroyuki Muta)

2 Characteristics of Movements and Activities in Patients with Parkinson's Disease

Troubles that Patients Have in Their Daily Lives

Patients with Parkinson's disease (PD) have motor symptoms such as tremors, rigidity, bradykinesia, posture and balance disorder. In addition, they have non-motor symptoms such as autonomic nervous system disorders and depression[1]. The presence of a higher brain function disorder in the early stages of PD has recently been determined[1,2]. However, a detailed description of the disorder the disease causes in their lives is not yet known. For example, contradictoriness movement (kinésie paradoxale)[3] such as "To freeze up on the level ground, but to be able to go up the stairs" occurs in walking and also in various circumstances. We investigated disorders of the everyday lives of patients with PD[4]. From interviews with 150 patients various characteristics were found.

Movements and Activities that Patients were used to Become Difficult

It is common for patients with PD to have difficulties in movements or activities they were used to doing. This occurs not only in "the walk" but also in self-care and domestic work. Patients had similar complaints: "cannot easily use chopsticks, a pencil or a kitchen knife," "putting on and taking off of clothes is not possible," and "it is not possible to clean and to cook." Some motor symptoms may influence these difficulties. However, there are difficulties thought to be caused by a higher brain function disorder[1,2]. Patients explained as follows: "The initial difficulties were strange symptoms. I could not hang a jacket on a hanger, and I could not take an object out of a bag"; "I cannot remember how to put my arm through a sleeve of a jacket"; "I cannot remember how to fold laundry," and so on. We analyzed various episodes that patients with PD talked about. As a result, the following characteristics could be determined.

1. **Movements or activities that are carried out unconsciously are difficult. When patients with PD consciously do movements or activities they can perform them.**

"I can use chopsticks when I am conscious of the correct grip and movement." "When I roll over and stand up I have to be conscious of the sequence of movements to move my hands, feet and body. If I start these movements without imaging them, I cannot do them." "When my gait suddenly freezes, I can begin to walk by imaging the several steps that I will need to take to get to the door or by imaging the direction of my foot when I step forward." "I can write letters and numbers as usual by first imaging that movement."

Patients with PD may have a decrease in ability to perform unconscious movements, and their coping method is to consciously perform movements and activities.

2. Why do patients have to perform movements and activities consciously?

When we drive a car or make meals the neural representation of action sequences and movement plans are already present before we carry out the actual activity. This process results from past movement learning. During the period that we learn to drive a car or make meals, this representation process is achieved because we consciously do the movements. However, while that learning gradually advances, it becomes possible for us to unconsciously and quickly do the same movements[3]. It is the basal ganglia and supplementary motor area in the brain that are strongly associated with our movement learning, unconscious representation of actions and movements, and execution of actions and movements[5,6].

PD is caused by a deficiency of dopamine due to the degeneration of the midbrain substantia nigra cells. Malfunction occurs in the basal ganglia because of dopamine deficiency. This results in the difficulty for patients with PD to perform movements or activities that they were unconsciously used to doing. How patients deal with these difficulties is to consciously perform movements or activities, as if they were being performed for the first time. However, even if movements are consciously performed, success varies among patients and is not consistent. This is because the patient's ability changes depending on the type of movement or activity and also by the situation and surroundings the patient is in.

3. Complicated movements or activities are difficult.

Complex behaviors, such as the following, are difficult compared to simple behaviors.

1) Movements or activities requiring a sequence of steps are difficult.

For example, when a patient go shopping, what the person do would be "I take out money from my wallet and put the change and a receipt into my wallet, and then carry a shopping bag." Therefore they use a coping strategy to take the time for each movement and also to simplify the procedure by using electronic money.

2) Movements or activities that require doing two things at the same time are difficult.

"It is difficult to grill fish while cooking another dish." "I cannot step forward while opening a door." "When I try to do two activities at the same time, I end up by stop doing both." The coping strategy that they use is to avoid doing simultaneous movements. They achieve success by doing one activity at a time.

3) **Movements and activities to be carried out with both hands are difficult.**

"When I wash my face or hair with both hands, I do not know why, but both my hands stop. It is possible to do it when I only use one hand." "I cannot screw the cap back onto a plastic bottle." "It is difficult to put a letter in an envelope or a document in a plastic folder. I try to be conscious about the movement of both hands." These are movements and activities that require coordinated work in the left and right hemisphere of the brain, mainly in the supplementary motor area. The coping strategy that patients use is to simplify the movement by using one hand and to be conscious about the movement of both hands.

4) **Alternating repetitive motions and activities are difficult.**

"When I brush my teeth, I cannot maintain rhythm. It is possible to focus on one direction, for instance just up or just down. It is easy to focus on one direction when I rub my body with a towel." These are examples of the alternating repetitive movement disorder. The coping method is to simplify the movements.

4. Presence or absence of visual information influences movement.

The abilities that patients with PD can perform are affected by the situation they are in. "When I eat with chopsticks, my hand suddenly stops when I lose sight of it around and between my lips." "When I put my hand behind me to pull up my trousers, my hand can reach my trousers, but then I don't know how to move." "I have difficulty with a turn when I walk, but when the course has a mark showing me where to go next, I can easily change direction." "Because I freeze up when it becomes dusk and the house becomes dim, I turn on all the lights in the house at night." "I cannot sense where my hands and feet are under my blanket. Therefore, I cannot move. I can move if I can see part of my hands and feet."

These examples show that the presence or absence of visual information strongly influences movements and activities. Furthermore, visual information about one's body influences the patient as well as visual information such as a mark on the wall or a line on the floor.

5. Why can they move or act if there is visual information?

The phenomenon "to freeze up on level ground, but to be able to go up the stairs" is known as contradictoriness movement (kinésie paradoxale). This phenomenon results from the estrangement of the internally guided movement system from the externally guided movement system[3,5,6]. Basal ganglia/supplementary motor area/prefrontal area is associated with the internally guided movement system. Cerebellum/parietal lobe/

premotor area is associated with the externally guided movement system. Usually, we adequately combine these two kinds of movement systems and accomplish a movement without freezing up.

For example, the following activities are combinations of movements using the two kinds of movement systems. We scoop food with a spoon and carry it to the mouth even though we lose its visual information around and between our lips. We can button up the front of a shirt (with visual information) as well as zip up the back of a dress (without visual information). Internally guided movements or activities become difficult in patients with PD. They cannot move well when visual information is insufficient, such as in darkness or under a blanket. Patients, therefore, use coping methods that rely on visual information: to step over a line and begin to walk; to straighten their posture by using a mark or a mirror; and also to turn on the lights in all the rooms. In other words, patients learn to cope with many difficulties resulting from their illness of their internally guided movement system by successfully using their externally guided movement system.

6. A change in visual information influences movement.

A change in visual information influences movement. "I often freeze up indoors, but it is easy to walk outdoors. I feel as if I have suddenly been freed." "When I move to a narrow place from a wide place, I freeze up." "Because a plastic shopping bag changes shape, it is hard for me to put things into it. But it is easy to put things in a square and solid shopping basket." "I can walk when there aren't other people around, but I cannot walk in a crowd. When people around me move, I stagger."

Constant visual information that patients are used to is necessary for patients[7].

7. A weakness in body schema and motor imagery may cause difficulties.

A change of visual information is one factor that causes difficulties. Patients cannot adequately integrate visual information with their self-physical information. Information they can see will help them with their movements. By what difficulties the patients say they have we can infer that the patient has weak body schema and motor imagery[8,9]. "I have a bad sense of distance. My chopsticks and spoon hit the edge of my mouth." "When I reach for the doorknob, I almost fall down." "When I open the door of the refrigerator, the door hits my body." "I cannot sit straight down on a bed or on a toilet seat." Some patients spoke of episodes that suggest they have a weakness in knowing how to move their bodies. "I cannot put my toothbrush in the right direction towards my teeth and gums." "When I shave, I don't know the angle to keep my razor." Some patients use the following coping methods: "First, I touch a door and furniture. I can move by touching with just one finger. It is necessary to touch something and also look before I begin to move." "When I sit down on a chair or a toilet seat, I can sit straight down if I first touch the seat." These coping methods closely resemble those that patients use in the dark to identify where their body is located in relation to their surrounding objects.

8. Gradually situations affect movement more. Movements and activities become uniform.

Patients continue their daily lives with several coping methods : using visual information; consciously performing movements or activities; and simplifying complex procedures. As the disease gradually progresses, however, patients are affected more by each situation they are in. Their ability to successfully complete a movement or activity greatly varies on whether they perform it in a familiar situation or not. "When I'm in an unfamiliar restroom and bath, I cannot move." "If the location of objects are changed even a little from their usual places, it becomes extremely difficult for me to move." Patients strive to maintain their movements and activities that they have been used to. In order to make this possible, it is necessary for them to keep a constant and familiar situation and environment.

9. Continuing to do usual movements is necessary. Relearning a movement is possible.

PD is a progressive disease, so it has been thought that the movements and activities of patients only get worse. Many comments from patients, however, indicate the importance of continuing to do movements and the possibility of relearning movements. "I continued teaching traditional Japanese dance even after getting PD. I don't feel the problem of posture and balance." "I began to move again by repeating an exercise." "The movement of my hand became so bad, that I gave up playing a musical instrument. Then I started practicing every single movement as if I were learning for the first time. I can now play on stage again." "I was good at knitting, but suddenly it became difficult. I practiced many times consciously being aware of how to move the needles and my fingers. Now I can knit as well as before."

Continuing a movement or activity is important to maintain the patient's abilities. Practice helps relearning a movement or activity that the patient finds difficult. The possibility of relearning a skill increases according to the frequency of having done that movement or activity in the past. In addition, for patients to relearn abilities that they once had requires gradual and careful repetition.

10. Other characteristic difficulties.

Many patients with PD spoke of pleasure-displeasure feelings and of moderate feelings of strain that affect their movements or activities. "I only feel a sense of safety when I see a handrail in a bathroom. My frozen gait is reduced." "When I feel unhappy, my movement really stops." "I cannot move when someone says something unpleasant to me." "Strangely enough, it is easy to get up when I am going to get something I like." "When I play my favorite sports, I can move without any problems." "It is easy for me to move when I am with people who I get along well with." "I feel moderate tension on a day at work, so I can move more easily than I do on my days off."

The basal ganglia has neural network between the limbic system as well as the brain cortex[3,10,11]. It is thought that this is the factor why the patients' psychological conditions and feelings have an influence on their movements.

Summary

The author describes the difficulties and characteristics of patients with PD. This information came from patients with PD. If this information helps improve other patients' daily lives, we are very happy. These findings, however, have yet to be scientifically validated. Future studies are still needed to help improve the everyday lives of patients.

(Shinichi Takabatake)

References

1) Otsuki M : Parkinson-Byou no Koujinoukinousyougai [Higher brain dysfunction in Parkinson's disease patients]. *MB Med Reha* **76** : 21-29, 2007 (in Japanese)
2) Uluduz D, et al : Apraxia in Parkinson's disease and multiple system atrophy. *Eur J Neurol* **17** : 413-418, 2010
3) Hikosaka O : Me to Seishin [Eyes and Mind]. Igaku-Shoin, pp86-168, 2003 (in Japanese)
4) Takabatake S, Tomatsu Y, Naito Y, et al : Parkinson-Byou Toujisya ni Okeru Nitijyouseikatsudousa no Konnan to Sono Tokusei [Difficulties in activities of daily living of patients with Parkinson's disease and its characteristics]. *Jpn J Osaka Occup Ther Assoc* **23** : 57-63, 2009 (in Japanese)
5) Tanji J : Nou to Undo [Brain and Action]. Kyoritsu-Shuppan, pp107-117, 1999 (in Japanese)
6) Tanji J : Nou no Koujikinou [Higher brain function]. Asakura Publishing Co. pp79-88, 2001 (in Japanese)
7) Higuchi T : Shintai Undogaku [Body Kinematics Message from Perception and Cognition]. Miwa-Shoten, pp124-147, 2008 (in Japanese)
8) Morioka S : Rehabilitation no Tameno Noshinkeigaku Nyumon [Basic Knowledge of Brain Functions and Neuroscience Useful for Rehabilitation]. Kyodo Isho-Shuppan, pp73-97, 2005 (in Japanese)
9) Iriki A : Dougu wo Tsukau Saru [Apes use tools, it is homo faber]. Igaku-Shoin, pp82-89, 2004 (in Japanese)
10) Takakusaki K : Dainoukiteikaku no Kinou [Function of the basal ganglia : associated with Parkinson's disease]. *J Physiol Soc Jpn* **65** (4, 5) : 113-129, 2003 (in Japanese)
11) Takakusaki K : Dainou Kiteikaku ni yoru Undo no Seigyo [The motor control by basal ganglia]. *Clinical Neurology* **49** (6) : 325-334, 2009 (in Japanese)

Part 2
Understanding Parkinson's Disease

1 Assessment of Parkinson's Disease

Functional Evaluation of Parkinson's Disease

In this chapter, we will discuss the functional evaluation indices of Parkinson's disease (PD) that are commonly used in the current clinical setting for different severity levels and for functions of the upper and lower extremities.

Severity Rating

Currently, the Hoehn and Yahr severity classification[1] and the Unified Parkinson's Disease Rating Scale (UPDRS)[2] are the most globally accepted rating scales for PD, and the Japanese versions of these are also widely used in Japan. Clinically, the simple and convenient Hoehn and Yahr severity classification is used to ascertain the general symptoms, and the UPDRS is used to evaluate the symptoms in greater detail. However, the UPDRS is not sufficient for evaluating diurnal variation of symptoms such as wearing off or delayed on, and a separate record such as a diary that reveals the changes within a day is required for such evaluations.

1. Hoehn and Yahr Severity Classification[1]

The Hoehn and Yahr scale classifies the severity level into five stages, I–V. The symptoms and manifestations of each stage are described below:

Stage I. Unilateral involvement only, usually with minimal or no functional impairment.

Stage II. Bilateral or midline involvement, without impairment of balance.

Stage III. First sign of impaired righting reflexes. This is evident by unsteadiness as the patient turns or is demonstrated when he is pushed from standing equilibrium with the feet together and eyes closed. Functionally the patient is somewhat restricted in his activities but may have some work potential depending upon the type of employment. Patients are physically capable of leading independent lives, and their disability is mild to moderate.

Stage IV. Fully developed, severely disabling disease; the patient is still able to walk and stand unassisted but is markedly incapacitated.

Stage V. Confinement to bed or wheelchair unless aided.

As described above, the classification of the stages is very simple and convenient, and it is heavily used as a method that illustrates the severity of disease (extent of progression) from the perspective of the patient's motor ability, since it is not affected by small changes in symptoms. In Japan, stage Ⅲ or greater in the Hoehn and Yahr severity classification (+degree of functional disability in daily life of Ⅱ-Ⅲ) is defined as the standard for the Research Project for the Treatment of Special Chronic Diseases of the Ministry of Health, Labour and Welfare. However, since it focuses on whether there is impairment in balance or activities of daily life, it is not suited for determining detailed treatment effects.

2．UPDRS (Unified Parkinson's Disease Rating Scale)[2)]

UPDRS consists of four parts with a total of 42 types of questions that are asked in 55 items. Parts Ⅰ through Ⅲ are evaluated on a 5-step scale from 0 (normal or no symptom) to 4 (severe), but seven items in Part Ⅳ are evaluated on a 2-step scale of 0 (no symptom) and 1 (with symptom). The maximum cumulative score from Part Ⅰ to Part Ⅳ is 199.

The descriptions of each of the four parts are as follows : Part Ⅰ evaluates mentation such as cognitive dysfunction, hallucinations, and depression, and consists of four items with a maximum total score of 16. Part Ⅱ evaluates the activities of daily living including speech, handwriting, eating, taking a bath, dressing, walking, and abnormal sensation, and consists of 13 items with a maximum total score of 52. Part Ⅲ evaluates the extent of PD symptoms in terms of motor function including speech, tremor, rigidity, postural reflex impairment, walking, and akinesia, and consists of 14 questions. Tremor at rest and rigidity are each evaluated in five items (the face/neck region, and in both upper and lower extremities), and postural tremor of the hands, finger tapping, opening and closing movements of hands, pronation-supination movements of the hands, and leg agility are evaluated in two items (both hands/legs). This sums up to 27 items in Part Ⅲ with a maximum total score of 108. Part Ⅳ evaluates the complications of therapy including dyskinesia, diurnal variation, and other complications, and seven of the 11 items are evaluated on a 2-step scale, either 0 (no) or 1 (yes). The maximum total score in this part is 23. This scale is most widely used currently because its validity and reliability have been proven in many studies. Although UPDRS has disadvantages in that it is time-consuming and is insufficient in evaluating symptom fluctuation and therapy complications, its reliability is high. Thus, it will most likely be used widely in the future as a PD rating scale.

Functional Evaluation

Traditionally, factors that inhibit the activities of daily living (ADL) in PD patients have been primarily viewed as motor function impairments that are caused by extrapyramidal symptoms, and rehabilitation has been conducted by mainly targeting the movement disorder caused by the four major symptoms (tremor, rigidity, akinesia/bradykinesia, and postural reflex impairment) of PD. With such a background in mind, typical indices that are clinically used for the functional evaluation of the four extremities will now be introduced by separating the evaluation into the functions of the upper and lower extremities.

1. Evaluation of upper extremity function

Tremor, rigidity, and akinesia/bradykinesia symptoms that impact the upper extremity function of PD patients include: impairment in voluntary movements caused by postural or action tremor; difficulties in performing rapid repetitive or intricate movements of the upper extremity with increasing severity; and delayed initiation of movements. Other symptoms are manifested as behavioral impairment, including clumsy handling of tools and difficulties in conventional movements; for example, problems are known to arise when patients perform common yet essential tasks such as buttoning clothes. Recently, there has been a series of reports that investigated these symptoms and determined them to be motor clumsiness or apraxia. Goldenberg et al.[3] tested for ideomotor apraxia (IMA) in PD patients and showed that they had decreased scores. Furthermore, they reported that their scores were not related to the severity of the movement disorder but were correlated with visuospatial and visuoperceptual abilities. Quencer et al.[4] conducted finger tapping and coin rotation tasks in PD patients and healthy controls, and they reported that limb-kinetic apraxia is associated with PD. In other words, there are opinions that conventional extrapyramidal symptoms including slowness of movement, tremor, and muscle rigidity cause movement difficulties in PD patients, but there is also the perspective that apraxia factors are associated with these symptoms. These reports suggest that, when evaluating the upper extremity function of PD patients, it is necessary to consider not only the decreased function caused by extrapyramidal symptoms such as tremor, rigidity, and akinesia/bradykinesia, but also impairment at the preparation stages of a movement.

Finger tapping and coin rotation tasks that test the finger operability, as well as the Simple Test for Evaluating Hand Function (STEF) that quantitatively measures the overall upper extremity function in PD patients, will be introduced.

1) Finger tapping

Finger tapping is also used in the UPDRS as an index that measures the speed of finger movements. The finger tapping method used by Quencer et al.[4] will be introduced.

The subjects are instructed to perform alternating movements of touching and releasing the tips of the thumb and index finger as rapidly as possible for ten seconds, and the number of taps is measured. The starting hand is chosen randomly, and tapping by each hand is measured three times, alternating between left and right.

Studies that quantitatively assessed finger tapping determined movement rhythm, maximum amplitude between fingers, and maximum speed in PD patients, and they found that the variability in rhythm was greater, the maximum amplitude between fingers was smaller, and the maximum speed tended to be slower in PD patients compared to healthy controls[5-7].

2) Coin rotation

Coin rotation has been used in recent years as a method that can easily and conveniently test the dexterity of finger movements. This test is considered to reflect coordination and dexterity of the fingers.

The method used by Quencer et al.[4] is described. The subjects rotate a coin 180° between their thumb, index finger, and middle finger as rapidly as possible for ten seconds, and the number of rotations is measured. Subjects are allowed to practice the task once per hand. The starting hand is selected randomly, and coin rotation by each hand is performed three times, alternating between left and right. The test is considered invalid and repeated if the subject drops the coin during the test.

To reiterate, Quencer et al.[4] conducted finger tapping and coin rotation tasks in PD patients and healthy controls, and they found that finger tapping was not different between the two groups, but coin rotation was significantly slower in PD patients. Furthermore, they demonstrated that the severity of PD was correlated with finger tapping but not with coin rotation. These results indicated that the clumsiness of PD patients demonstrated via the coin rotation task is different from the extrapyramidal disorder evaluated by the finger tapping task, and it is associated with limb-kinetic apraxia. Gebhardt et al.[8] conducted finger tapping and coin rotation tasks in PD patients when they were in ON or OFF medication states and compared their results with those of healthy controls. Although both finger tapping and coin rotation scores were significantly lower in the PD group in the OFF-state compared to healthy controls, the finger tapping score improved in the ON-state to a similar level to healthy controls. In contrast, coin rotation did not improve in the ON-state and remained significantly slower compared to healthy controls. This report also corroborated the interpretation that, in PD patients, the finger tapping score is affected by slowness of movement, while the coin rotation score is affected by elements other than slowness of movement.

From the above previous studies, the degree of deviation in finger tapping and the coin rotation results are predicted to demonstrate the degree of difficulty in preparing for upper extremity movements in PD patients.

Nonetheless, the validity and reliability of these tests that determined the extent in which upper extremity function decreased in PD patients have yet to be investigated, and future studies are anticipated to resolve this issue.

3) Simple Test for Evaluating Hand Function (STEF)[9,10]

The STEF measures the time required to move objects on a desk and objectively evaluates the movement ability of the upper extremity, especially the speed of movement. It is an evaluation index that is widely used in clinical occupational therapy. This test is used in patients with peripheral nerve injury, mild cerebrovascular disorder, dementia, and PD.

The test consists of ten types of subtests. The subjects are asked to perform a series of movements to hold, move, and release ten types of objects with different sizes, shapes, weights, and materials (baseball, building block, wooden disk, cloth, coin, pin, etc.) on the examination table. Each subtest is scored from 1-10 depending on the profile of time required to perform the task, and the total score from 1-100 is calculated for each hand.

The normal range is presented in 17 different age groups from "3 years old" to "80 years old," and the test can determine to what extent the subjects are limited in terms of the speed of their upper extremity movements. It can also compare the results with healthy controls. Since the results can be expressed quantitatively, the test is easy to use and explain to the patient and family, as well as to individuals working in other occupations. Each subtest has a time limit of 30-70 seconds, and the test is conducted in under 20 minutes.

Preparation of the test, processing of test data, and analysis of test results can also be completed in a short amount of time. This is one of the very few indices that can quantitatively determine upper extremity function with reliability and validity.

One of the issues with this test is that it cannot evaluate and verify the coordinated movements of both hands because there are no subtests that involve both hands. Since PD patients often complain of impairment in coordinated movements with both hands, such as "I cannot form rice balls with my hands" or "I cannot put bills in my wallet," we recognize that it is essential to evaluate the assessment methods.

2. Evaluation of lower extremity function

In addition to the movement disorder caused by the four major symptoms, in terms of lower extremity function, it is suggested that PD patients have difficulty at the preparation stages of a movement, such as being able to step forward with rhythmic sounds or visual stimulation (a marker).

The Timed Up and Go test (TUG), which is a representative assessment of dynamic balance and is also a comprehensive evaluation of lower extremity function, is introduced.

Timed Up and Go test (TUG) (Figure 1)[11,12]

The TUG can measure the ability to perform a series of movements that are incorporated in daily life, such as standing up, walking, changing direction, and sitting down. In other words, one of the features of this test is that it can evaluate the dynamic lower extremity function under conditions that are similar to actual daily life situations. Furthermore, this test can evaluate the muscle strength and the coordinated muscle activity

Figure 1 Timed Up and Go Test (TUG)
From the front legs of the chair To the distal part of the marker
3 m

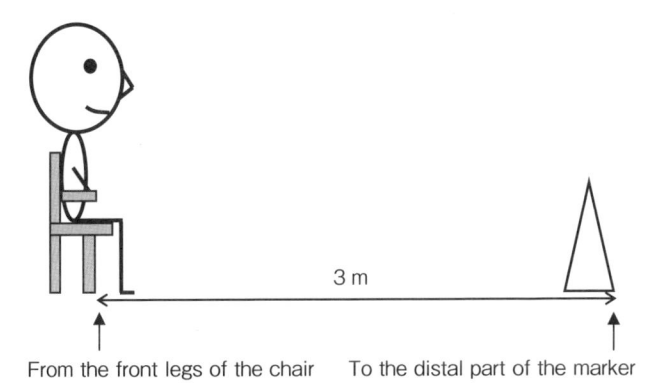

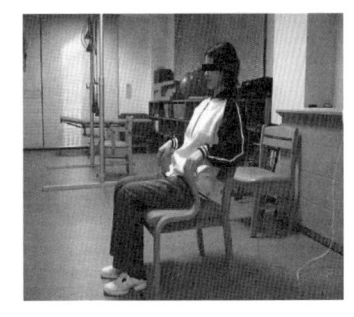

Figure 2 Starting Position

of the lower extremity and trunk, as well as the righting reflexes required to smoothly change directions and the ability to support or control lower extremities. Needless to say, it can also qualitatively assess propulsion, as well as difficulties in initiating movements and changing directions through observations.

【Method】
1. The subject sits in an armchair with his/her back resting on the back of the chair (**Figure 2**).
2. When the examiner gives the signal (the examiner says "Go" in the original version; in Japan, the examiner may say "Yo-i Don" which translates to "Get set, go") the subject will stand up, walk forward at a "comfortable" pace to the marker line three meters ahead, turn around, walk back to the chair, and sit down.
3. The subject is given instructions on this task and practices once. Once the subject fully understands the method, the test is performed.
4. The examiner measures the time required for the subject to perform a set of these movements.

The reliability and validity of this test have also been thoroughly investigated.

Podsiadlo et al.[11] presented criteria in the elderly who do not have abnormal motor function: the patient is capable if he/she performs the task within 10 seconds; the patient is considered to be able to go outside if the task is completed within 20 seconds; and the patient is considered to be at the level of requiring assistance if the task takes 30 seconds or longer to complete. Okubo et al.[13] investigated the association between the TUG and a history of multiple falls in PD patients who have trouble with everyday walking, and they reported that TUG time was significantly longer in those who have fallen multiple times compared to those who have not fallen, indicating that the TUG is an index associated with the risk for multiple falls. The above findings suggest that the TUG can be used as an index to assess the risk of falling in PD.

(Yasuo Naito)

References

1) Hoehn MM, et al : Parkinsonism: onset, progression and mortality. *Neurology* 17 : 427-442, 1967
2) Fahn S, et al : Unified Parkinson's Disease Rating Scale. In Fahn S, et al (eds) : Recent Developments in Parkinson's Disease. Vol II. Macmillan Healthcare Information, pp153-163, 293-305, 1987
3) Goldenberg G, et al : Impairment of motor planning in patients with Parkinson's disease: evidence from ideomotor apraxia testing. *J Neurol Neurosurg Psychiatry* 49 : 1266-1272, 1986
4) Quencer K, et al : Limb-kinetic apraxia in Parkinson disease. *Neurology* 68 : 150-151, 2007
5) Kandori A, et al : Quantitative magnetic detection of finger movements in patients with Parkinson's disease. *Neurosci Res* 49 : 253-260, 2004
6) Shima K, et al : Ningen no Yubi Tap Undoukeisoku wo Mokuteki to shita Jiki Sensor no Kakuseihou 〔A New Calibration Method of Magnetic Sensors for Measurement of Human Finger Tapping Movements〕. *Trans Soc Instrum Control Eng* 43 : 821-828, 2007 (in Japanese)
7) Okuno R, et al : Yubi Tap Kasokudo Keisoku System no Kaihatsu to Parkinson-Byou Shindan Shien eno Ohyo〔Development of a Finger-tapping Acceleration Measurement System for Quantitative Diagnosis of Parkinson's Disease〕. *Trans Jpn Soc Med Biol Eng* 43 : 752-761, 2005 (in Japanese)
8) Gebhardt A, et al : Poor dopaminergic response of impaired dexterity in Parkinson's disease—bradykinesia or limb kinetic apraxia? *Mov Disord* 23 : 1701-1706, 2008
9) Kaneko T : Kanni Jyoshi Kinou Kensa 〔Simple Test for Evaluating Hand Function (STEF) —Mannual〕. Sakai Med Co., 1986 (in Japanese)
10) Kanenari K, et al : Rehab ni okeru Outcome Hyoka Shakudo 〔Simple Test for Evaluating Hand Function (STEF), Manual Function Test (MFT)〕. *J Clin Rehabil* 15 : 470-474, 2006 (in Japanese)
11) Podsiadlo D, et al : The Timed "Up & Go" —a test of basic functional mobility for frail elderly persons. *J Am Geriatr Soc* 39 : 142-148, 1991
12) Mathias S, et al : Balance in elderly patients—the "Get-Up and Go" Test. *Arch Phys Med Rehabil* 67 : 387-389, 1986
13) Okubo S, et al : Hoehn & Yahr Stage 3, 4 no Parkinson-Byo Kanjya ni okeru Timed Up & Go Test to Fukusuukai Tentou tono Kankei 〔Relationship for Timed Up & Go Test and Fall in Parkinson's disease patients〕. *Nara Rigakuryouhougaku* 2 : 6-9, 2010 (in Japanese)

2 Assessment of Parkinson's Disease
Assessment of Body Schema Manuscript

Body Schema

1) Body Schema and Body Image

Body schema is a concept developed from the study of postural schema by Henry Head and Gordon Holmes[1]; Head and Holmes hypothesized the existence of an internal postural model that ensures smooth movement of the body by comparing postures or positions of the body before and after a movement has been performed. Additionally, the body schema is updated accordingly with these changes in posture and position of the body[2-4].

Paul Schilder[5] further advanced the concept of body schema from a psychological perspective by considering the effects of emotions and assumptions on body movement, thus developing the notion of body image[2,6-9], which he defined as "the image of the human body means the picture of our own body which we form in our mind"[5].

Although the terms "body schema" and "body image" have been used interchangeably on occasion, they are generally regarded as two distinct ideas because the latter has historically evolved from the former[10,11]. Despite this distinction, the two are not completely independent of each other; rather, they are closely related, in the sense that body image, formed in the consciousness, is rooted in and grows out of the body schema[12,13].

2) Three Types of Body Representation Functions

In recent years, the functions of body representations have at times been classified into three types: a) semantic and lexical representations, b) visual-spatial representations, and c) online representations[14-19].

a) Semantic and lexical representations refer to anatomical knowledge about the body as well as semantic and terminological information about body functions. Put simply, these pertain to people's knowledge of their own body parts, such as the names and functions.

b) Visual-spatial representations are body perceptions based mainly on visual information and specify locations of surface parts of the body as well as boundaries between the respective parts. These concern knowledge about body structures, including the shapes, areas, and spatial relations of body parts.

　c) Online representations are body coordination systems that process one's present posture three-dimensionally and dynamically on a real-time basis using various sensory information (e.g., deep and vestibular sensations) and efferent feedbacks at the moment when a change in body posture or position occurs within the external space.

　When compared to traditional classifications of body schema and body image, the idea of online representations almost coincide with that of body schema, while the concepts of semantic and lexical, and visual-spatial representations correspond to those of body image[20].

Body Schema Assessment Methods

Research on Parkinson's disease (PD) patients has indicated that these individuals' body representation functions show particular difficulties in processing body schema (especially online representations). Therefore, methods for assessing body schema (or online representations) are introduced here, classified into three main groups: sensory tests, imitation tasks, and drawing methods.

　Although several of these were designed for use with children (toddlers to school-aged), including sensory processing/praxis tests such as the Japanese Playful Assessment for Neuropsychological Abilities (JPAN)[21], we consider them to also be applicable to adult patients with PD and worth noting here.

1) Sensory Tests

(a) In-Between Test[22]

This was originally designed as a tactile test primarily to detect peripheral anesthesia. However, as tactility is a component of somatic sensation, which forms body schema, the test is considered an appropriate measure of body schema, as well.

【Method】

The subject is instructed to close his/her eyes and put his/her palm down on a desk. The examiner then touches two of the subject's fingers simultaneously. Then, the subject is asked to tell the number of fingers between the two that were touched. The same procedure is performed four times with each hand.

(b) Two-Point Finger Test[22]

Similar to the In-Between Test, this test was originally developed to evaluate tactility, but has been considered applicable to the assessment of body schema.

【Method】

The subject is requested to close his/her eyes and put his/her palm down on a desk. The examiner touches two spots on the subject's finger or fingers simultaneously. The subject is then asked to indicate if those two spots were on the same or different fin-

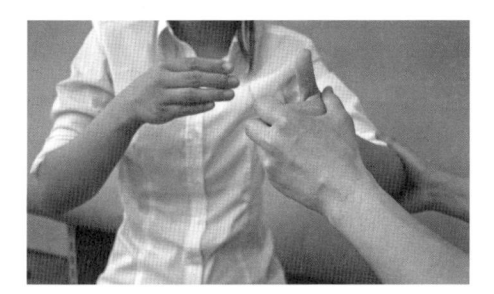

Figure Find the Thumb Test

gers. The same procedure is performed four times with each hand.

(c) Name the Finger Game[23]

This is one of the subscales of the JPAN test; this game consists of three parts, one of which measures visual-spatial representations (Part 1), while the other two assess body schema (or online representations; Parts 2 and 3).

【Method】

In Part 1, the examiner points to a finger on a hand pictured on a card. The subject is asked to feel his/her own hand and locate the corresponding finger while his/her hand is shielded from view. In Part 2, the examiner touches one of the subject's fingers when his/her hand is visually blocked. The subject is then asked to name the finger touched by the examiner. In Part 3, the examiner touches the subject's fingers in a sequence. The subject is asked to name the touched fingers in the same order.

(d) Find the Thumb Test[24,25]

This test evaluates the ability to recognize the spatial positions of one's thumbs. Because the test's validity has been established with regard to detecting dysfunction in proprioceptive sensation (which also forms body schema), it can be used in body schema assessments, too.

【Method】

The examiner grasps the subject's hand with one hand and covers all of the subject's fingers except for the thumb. With his/her free hand, the examiner holds the subject's arm at around the elbow and fixes it in the air.

Then, the examiner instructs the subject to grasp the thumb of his/her fixed hand with his/her other hand while the subject's eyes are open. After confirming that the subject can grasp the thumb properly, the examiner instructs the subject to close his/her eyes. Once again, the examiner holds the subject's arm and fixes it in place after moving it. The subject is again asked to try grasping the thumb of his/her fixed hand in the same manner as when his/her eyes are open.

The same procedure is performed several more times, after which the results are integrated for assessment (**Figure**).

2) Imitation Tasks

(a) Imitation of Limb Posture

This is a subordinate test of the Southern California Sensory Integration Test (SCSIT)[26]. The task is considered to involve body schema (or online representations) and visual-spatial representations.

【Method】

The subject and examiner sit face-to-face on armless chairs. The subject is instructed to take the same posture as the examiner. The examiner takes twelve postures, utilizing both his/her upper and lower limbs, including the fingers. The examiner maintains each posture for ten seconds or until the subject succeeds in taking the correct posture.

    The subject scores 2 points if he/she takes the correct posture within three seconds, and scores 1 if he/she takes the correct posture after four seconds but within ten seconds. If the subject takes the correct posture only after ten seconds or if his/her posture is not correct, he/she receives a "0".

(b) "Let's Mimic and Be Cool"[27]

This imitation task, a part of the JPAN, assesses body schema (or online representations) and visual-spatial representations.

【Method】

The examiner shows an illustration (a photo of a child striking a pose) and asks the subject to imitate the child's pose in the picture. The examiner and subject stand face-to-face, with a space of about one and a half meters between them (so that the subject can see the illustration clearly).

3) Drawing Methods

(a) "Let's Play in the Park"[28]

This is a JPAN test item. This task provides an integrated measure of a person's abilities to use the three types of representations in processing body schema: semantic, visual-spatial, and online.

【Method】

The subject is instructed to draw pictures of a person in the following positions: (a) standing at an entrance of a park (standing), (b) hanging from a horizontal bar (horizontal bar), (c) sitting on a chair (chair), and (d) crawling on his/her stomach in a tunnel (crawling). Drawing tasks (a) and (b) are obligatory, while tasks (c) and (d) are regarded as referential tests for more in-depth assessment.

Regarding Body Schema Assessment Methods

Because body schema is updated continuously online from constant and various input of sensory information, including deep sensations, it is considered difficult to assess with a single test or task. Body schema must be interpreted comprehensively or multi-dimensionally according to the results of more than one test or task that is specifically designed to fully capture the various elements of body schema.

In the field of occupational therapy, few references appear to have been made thus far concerning methods assessing body schema, though the importance of such assessments has often been noted. In the future, development of a specialized body schema assessment scale for occupational therapy is expected.

(Hiroaki Tanaka)

References

1) Head H, Holmes G : Sensory disturbances from cerebral lesions. *Brain* 34 : 102-254, 1911
2) Ohigashi Y : Shintai Zushiki [Body Schema]. Iwanami Koza Seishin no Kagaku 4 : Seishin to Shintai [Iwanami Lecture Science of Mind 4 : Mind and Body]. Iwanami-Shoten, pp 209-236, 1983 (in Japanese)
3) Hashimoto T, et al : Jiko Shintaizo Ninchi [Own body representation]. *Molecular Psychiatry* 11 : 71-72, 2011 (in Japanese)
4) Sakata H : Tochoyo no Hakai Shojo [Damaged Conditions of Frontal Lobe]. In Sakata H, et al : Tochoyo [Frontal Lobe]. Igaku-Shoin, pp 73-101, 2006 (in Japanese)
5) Schilder P (author), Inenaga K (ed.) : Shintai no Shinrigaku [Psycology of the Body], Seiwa-Shoten, pp 278-327, 1987 (in Japanese)
6) Kono T : ＜Kokoro＞wa Karada no Soto ni Aru [＜Heart＞is Outside the Body]. NHK Publishing Inc., pp 187-211, 2006 (in Japanese)
7) Saiganji H : Shintai Image [Body Image]. Iwanami Koza Seishin no Kagaku 4 : Seishin to Shintai [Iwanami Lecture Science of Mind 4 : Mind and Body]. Iwanami-Shoten, pp 177-208, 1983 (in Japanese)
8) Blakeslee S, et al (author), Komatsu J (translation) : No no Naka no Shintai Chizu [Body Map in the Brain]. Intershift, pp 45-86, 2007
9) Schilder P (Author), Hojo K (translation) : Shintai Zushiki [Body Schema]. Kongo-Shuppan, pp 125-146, 1983
10) Tanaka S : Shintai Image no Tetsugaku [Philosophy of Body Image]. *Clini Neurosci* 29 : 868-871, 2011 (in Japanese)
11) Gallagher S : How the body shapes the mind, Oxford University Press, pp 17-39, 2005
12) Higuchi T : Shintai to Kukan no Hyosho [Representations of Body and Space]. In Higuchi T, et al (authors) : Shintai Undogaku [Body Kinematics]. Miwa-Shoten, pp 107-147, 2008 (in Japanese)
13) Yamane H : Chiryo/Enjo ni Okeru Futatsu no Communication [Two Communications in Treatment and Support]. Miwa-Shoten, pp 24-27, 2008 (in Japanese)
14) Sirigu A, et al : Multiple representations contribute to body knowledge processing. *Brain* 114 : 629-642, 1991
15) Coslett HB : Evidence for a disturbance of the body schema in neglect. *Brain Cogn* 37 : 527-544, 1998
16) Coslett HB, et al : Knowledge of the human body—A distinct semantics domain. *Neurology* 59 : 357-363, 2002
17) Schwoebel J, et al : Evidence for multiple, distinct representations of the human body. *J Cogn Neurosci* 17 : 543-553, 2005
18) Tsuruya N, et al : Ryosokutochoyo Ishuku to Jikoshintaibui Shitsunin [Bilateral Parietal Lobe Atrophy and Autotoagnosia]. *Clini Neurosci* 27 : 403-406, 2009 (in Japanese)

19) Tsuruya N : Jikoshintaibui Shitsunin [Autotoagnosia]. *Neuropsychology* 27 : 304-314, 2011 (in Japanese)
20) de Vignemont F : Body schema and body image—Pros and cons. *Neuropsychologia* 48 : 669-680, 2010
21) The Japanese Academy of Sensory Integration (ed) : JPAN Kankakushori/Koui Kinokensa Jissi Manual [Sensory Processing/Praxis Tests : Implementation Manual], Pacific Supply Co. Ltd., pp 24-30, 2011 (in Japanese)
22) Akiyama T : Body Image. Agari I (ed) : Shinri Assessment Handbook. 2nd ed.[Psychological Assessment Handbook 2nd ed]. Nishimura shoten Co. Ltd., pp 516-528, 1993 (in Japanese)
23) The Japanese Academy of Sensory Integration (ed) : JPAN Kankakushori/Koui Kinokensa Jissi Manual [Sensory Processing/Praxis Tests : Implementation Manual], Pacific Supply Co. Ltd., pp 44-47, 2011 (in Japanese)
24) Hirayama K : Boshi Sagashi Shiken [Find the Thumb Test]. *Clinical Neurology* 26 : 448-454, 1986 (in Japanese)
25) Nakata M, et al : Chikaku wo Miru/Ikasu [See and utilize perception]. Kyodo Isho-Shuppan Co. Ltd., pp 51-53, 2003 (in Japanese)
26) Ayres AJ : Southern California Sensory Integration Tests. Western Psychological Services, 1972
27) The Japanese Academy of Sensory Integration (ed) : JPAN Kankakushori/Koui Kinokensa Jissi Manual [Sensory Processing/Praxis Tests : Implementation Manual], Pacific Supply Co. Ltd., pp 60-62, 2011 (in Japanese)
28) The Japanese Academy of Sensory Integration (ed) : JPAN Kankakushori/Koui Kinokensa Jisshi Manual [Sensory Processing/Praxis Tests : Implementation Manual], Pacific Supply Co. Ltd., pp 94-100, 2011 (in Japanese)

3 Assessment of Parkinson's Disease
Evaluation of Motor Imagery

Motor Imagery

It is considered that motor imagery is a movement rehearsal to recall the movement without actually performing of the movement, which is a cognitive process that is regenerated in the working memory in the brain[1]. Motor imagery plays an important role in order to perform the movements efficiently in life. For example, the way of holding a cup of cold water differs from that of a hot coffee, though both cups have no difference in shape and figure. In the case of the cold cup, we catch it with all fingers. On the other hand, in the case of the hot cup, we do it in the way of lessening the contact surface. Even if we cannot hold the cup, we may be able to plan appropriate performance of the movement on the base of visual information. Such a planning performed mentally without any motor output is regarded as a motor imagery that is a cognitive process.

Since studies of Roland et al.[2] in the 1980s, motor imagery has become to be noticed. They reported that the cerebral blood flows in the premotor cortex and supplementary motor area were increased when recalling the movement of the opposition of the thumb and the rest of fingers in Positron Emission Tomography (PET). Jackson et al.[3] reported that the similar regions in the brain activated in the actually performing of the movement and recalling of motor imagery. Weinrich et al.[4] have reported that the activities of the premotor cortex and supplementary motor area have preceded actually performing of movements. In other words, a motor imagery recalling is carried out in *advance* of the actually performing of the movement, and in only imaging, premotor cortex and supplementary motor area become to be activated. In recent years, the development of instrumentation has been to enable to study brain activities on motor imagery in various diseases and brain activities prior to movements or its impairment draw researchers' attention.

Evaluation of Motor Imagery

It is said that quantification or evaluation of motor imagery is difficult because it is not visible and is a cognitive process. The following three methods can be usually used as simple methods for evaluating the motor imagery ability.

1. Mental chronometry test

The mental chronometry test is a method for comparing the imagined time with the real time of performing movements[5]. It is considered that the nearer both of the time are, the higher motor recalling imagery ability is. It can be applied to various movements, but there is a problem that the criterion is not clear because a unified way has not been established.

2. Questionnaire method

Questionnaire method is intended to measure the clarity of imaging, using a questionnaire. It is a technique that has been developed in sport psychological fields. In order to evaluate the subjective easiness of imaging, Hall et al.[6] created the Movement Imagery Questionnaire-revised (MIQ-R). In Japan, Hasegawa[7] created the Movement Imagery Questionnaire-revised Japanese version (JMIQ-R) based on the MIQ-R. JMIQ-R consisting of eight items entailing visually or kinesthetically imaging that movement assesses each clarity of movements on a point scale from 1 to 7. By referring to the MIQ-R, the Kinesthetic and Visual Imagery Questionnaire (KVIQ) has been made for the elderly and the handicapped[8]. This test is easy to use because the method has been unified, but there is a problem that the score points may be changeable depending on the degree of understanding of the question when answering the subjective easiness of generating that image.

3. Mental Rotation task

Mental Rotation task is designed to test how accurately and rapidly the subject, who is shown limbs and figures which are rotated a specific amount of degrees, can distinguish between the mirrored and non-mirrored pairs and between the rotated and non-rotated pairs[9]. It is said that the shorter the time to answer is, the higher motor imagery ability is. It is easy to use clinically because it can be tested in a short time, but there is a problem that the criterion is not clear because a unified way has not been established.

Motor Imagery of Parkinson's Disease Patients

In the study of the motor image of Parkinson's disease (PD) patients, Heremans et al.[10] compared 14 patients with PD with 14 healthy subjects on the imagery ability using KVIQ and MIQ. They reported that there was no difference in the imagery ability between the two groups.

Amick et al.[11] made an investigation of 12 PD patients with severe impairment on the left side, 15 PD patients with severe impairment on the right side and 13 healthy subjects, using the Mental Rotation task—hand and block. No difference was observed

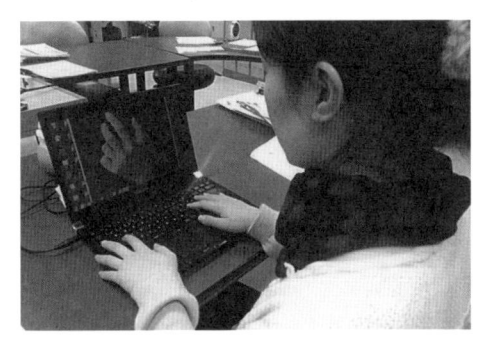

Figure 1 Mental Rotation task

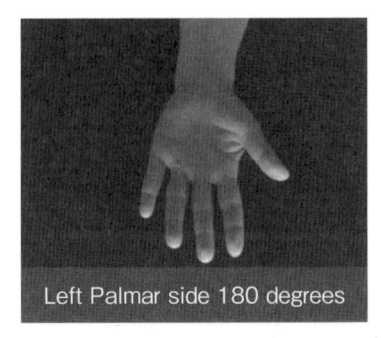

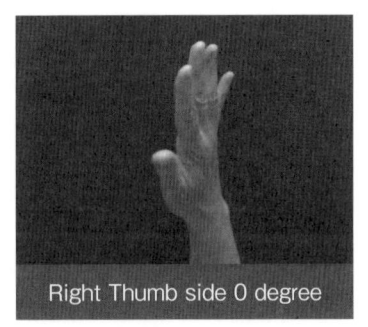

Figure 2 Pieces of the Hand

in the three groups on the block task. In the Mental Rotation task on the hand task, however, they reported that patients with severe impairment on the right side have made more errors than healthy subjects.

We will report findings of motor imagery in PD patients, which were obtained from the investigation using a Mental Rotation task of distinguishing the left hand from the right hand.

1. Mental Rotation task of the hand

We adopted the task of distinguishing the left hand from the right hand as a Mental Rotation task in this study. We displayed tasks for subjects on the screen of the personal computer (**Figure 1**). It consisted of 48 pieces of the hand which were the three kinds of photographs taken from the thumb side, dorsal side, and the palmar side of the hand and rotated to eight directions of every 45 degrees (**Figure 2**). The correct answer rate and reaction time to answer was recorded.

2. Comparison between PD patients and healthy subjects

1) Methods

Normal group : 48 people (11 males and 37 females)

They could answer with language without cognitive impairment symptoms and any

Table Reaction Time

	PD patients (n=21)	Healthy subjects (n=48)	p value	Significance level
reaction time (s)[a]	169.89±78.98	101.47±26.73	p<0.001	**

U-test of Mann-Whitney, [a]Mean ± SD, **p<0.001

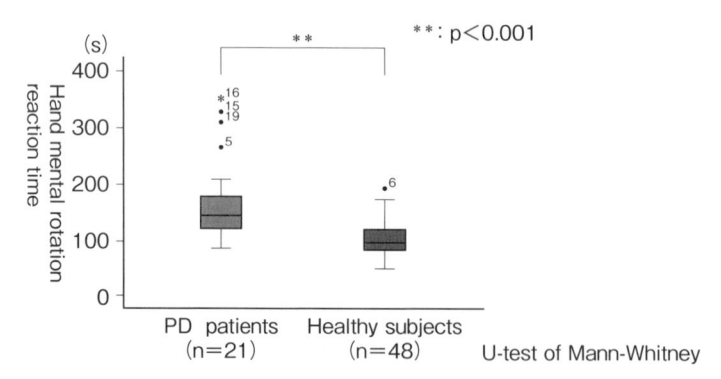

Figure 3 Hand Mental Rotation Reaction Time

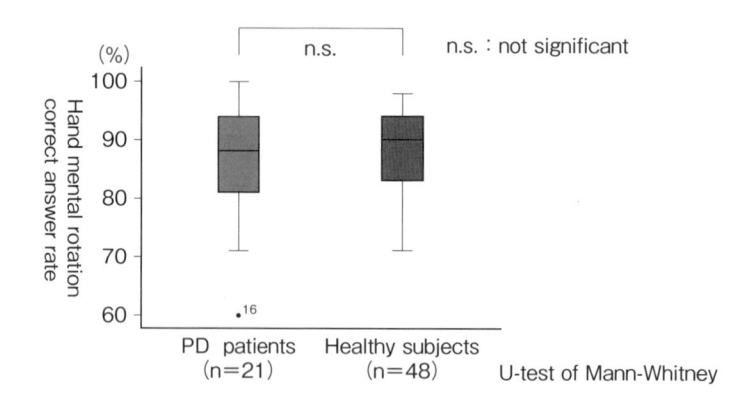

Figure 4 Hand Mental Rotation Correct Answer Rate

neurological abnormalities that affect this study.

PD patients: 21 patients (7 males and 14 females)

①Diagnosis was confirmed.

②They could answer with language without cognitive impairment symptoms.

③There was no abnormal neurological deficits that affect this study, except for PD.

④21 PD patients who were classified in Ⅰ-Ⅴ Hoehn & Yahr severity classification could operate upper limbs in sitting position.

⑤Each subject who had stable symptoms without alternation of medication until a month just before this study, was also compared and discussed in consideration of age or sex.

Analysis:

The reaction times to answer were compared with the correct answer rate by using the

U-test of Mann-Whitney.

2) Results

The reaction times were longer in PD patients in comparison with healthy subjects. A significant difference was observed between the groups (Table, Figure 3).

There was no significant difference on the correct answer rate between the two groups (Figure 4).

3) Discussion

The motor imagery abilities were decreased in PD patients. However, the correct answer rate was not decreased.

Namely, although patients with PD take more time to recall motor imagery, we believe that their motor imageries are correct.

Summary

In this chapter, we presented the results of our studies, a little reviews of literatures in PD, each way of Mental Rotation task, questionnaire and mental chronometry as the evaluation of motor imagery ability. Currently, the evaluation of motor imagery has been performed for orthopedic diseases, stroke and PD. The matters of motor planning have become to be obvious.

However, a unified method of how to evaluate has not been established. Different ways of evaluation have been executed in every study, finally, it is desirable that a unified method develops moreover in the future.

(Hajime Nakanishi, Fumika Makio, Hideki Miyaguchi)

References

1) Decety J : The neurophysiological basis of motor imagery. *Behav Brain Res* 77 : 45-52, 1996
2) Roland PE, et al : Supplementary motor area and other cortical areas in organization of voluntary movements in man. *J Neurophysiol* 43 : 118-136, 1980
3) Jackson PL, et al : Potential role of mental practice using motor imagery in neurologic rehabilitation. *Arch Phys Med Rehabil* 82 : 1133-1141, 2001
4) Weinrich M, et al : A neurophysiological study of the premotor cortex in the rhesus monkey. *Brain* 107 : 385-414, 1984
5) Malouin F, et al : Reliability of mental chronometry for assessing motor imagery ability after stroke. *Arch Phys Med Rehabil* 89 : 311-319, 2008
6) Hall CR, et al : Measuring movement imagery abilities—a revision of the movement imagery questionnaire. *J Ment Imagery* 21 : 143-154, 1997
7) Hasegawa N : Nihon ban Undo Shinsyo Shitsumon-shi Kaitei ban (JMIQ-R) no Sakusei [The development of a Japanese Version of the Revised Movement Imagery Questionnaire]. *The Japanese Journal of Mental Imagery* 2 : 25-34, 2004 (in Japanese)
8) Malouin F, et al : The Kinesthetic and Visual Imagery Questionnaire (KVIQ) for assessing motor imagery in persons with physical disabilities: a reliability and construct validity study. *J Neurol Phys Ther* 31 : 20-29, 2007
9) Parsons LM, et al : Cerebrally lateralized mental representations of hand shape and

movement. *J Neurosci* 18：6539-6548, 1998
10) Heremans E, et al：Motor imagery ability in patients with early- and mid-stage Parkinson disease. *Neurorehabil Neural Repair* 25：168-177, 2011
11) Amick MM, et al：Frontostriatal circuits are necessary for visuomotor transformation—mental rotation in Parkinson's disease. *Neuropsychologia* 44：339-349, 2006

Part 3

Neurodance-Exercise for People with Parkinson's Disease

1 Elements and Structure of the Dance Programs for Parkinson's Disease

Introduction

The rehabilitation program for Parkinson's disease (PD) is mainly for the improvement of movement at present, and one for either cognitive functions or mental symptoms has not been established[1]. We (PD study group) considered that, regarding the rehabilitation for PD, it is important to approach this problem by understanding the reasons of PD patients' difficulty in daily living from their brain functions. Because cognitive dysfunctions and mental symptoms often greatly affect their daily living[2], we made a dance program, called "Neurodance" as a part of a rehabilitation program that can involve motor and cognitive functions, and mental symptoms at the same time.

Dance programs for PD patients have started to attract attention abroad. In the United States, dance groups for PD patients have been organized under the guidance of dancers and they offer dance classes based on the patients' imagined movements[3]. In Argentina, it has been found that the quick turns of tango and dancing in pairs are very effective against PD[4]. We are offering dance classes to the patients with PD based on these previous studies. The participants often say "Recently, my walking pace has become fast," "I can do things more quickly," and "I participate in other activities, too." These changes suggest that dance programs are effective for improving movement, cognitive functions and mental symptoms.

This chapter proposes a hypothesis about the effectiveness of dance on the improvement of the cognitive function of PD patients based on its characteristics, and at the same time, it explains the important parts of the elements and structure considered to be important for the dance program.

Characteristics of PD and Structure of the Neurodance (Figure 1)

PD is due to the breakdown of interaction with the frontal cortex caused by the degeneration of basal ganglia, so that it develops cognitive dysfunctions (procedural learning disorder, procedural memory disorder, executive function disorder, and effective memory utilization disorder)[5]. The strategies of rehabilitation for these cognitive dysfunctions are thought to consist of methods such as "focus," "practice decomposed movement into simple parts," "repeat practice," "perform a mental rehearsal," and "utilize

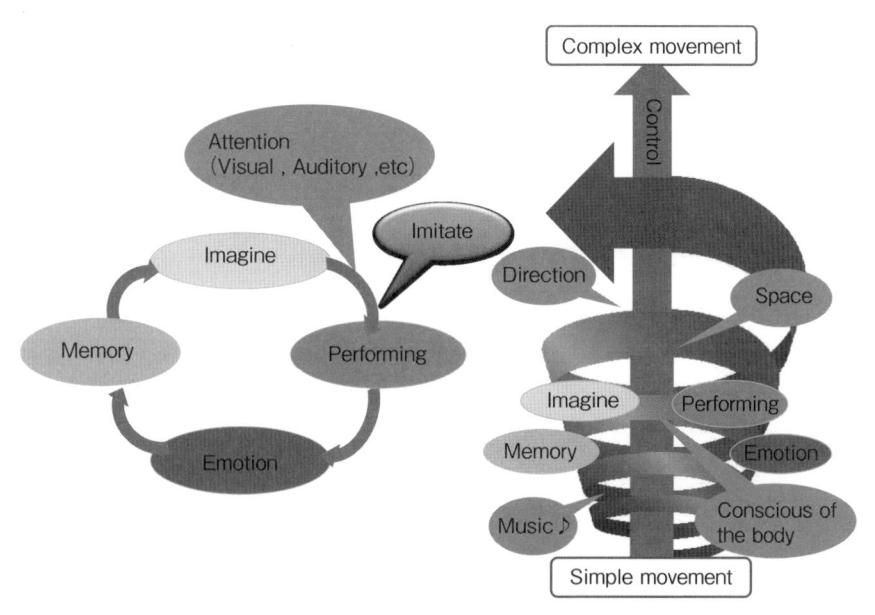

Figure 1　Structure of the Neurodance

cues" [6-7]. It also includes functional recoveries such as neuronal reconnection and functional compensation using external cues and an internal memory strategy[8]. One of the characteristics of the dance is the improvement of cognitive functions by planning and performing the imagined motion using movements such as physical flexibility, the speed and balance of movements and steps, moving in time to music and cues, memorizing the movements by repeating them, and gaining consciousness of oneself. Another characteristic is the improvement of mental symptoms by the enjoyment of moving the body to rhythm. These characteristics of dance play strategic roles in the rehabilitation of motor dysfunctions and cognitive dysfunctions and, at the same time, involve mental symptoms. Dance is certainly one intervention method to comprehensively improve the deteriorated functions caused by PD.

Elements Necessary for the PD Dance (Figure 2)

The movements and elements necessary for the PD dance were considered from characteristics of the difficulties that PD patients have in daily activities and their ways in approaching these difficulties.

The characteristics of PD patients in daily living are: 1) difficulty in moving in a condition of no visual information; 2) difficulty in moving in a complex way; 3) difficulty in unconscious movements; 4) difficulty in quick switch of movements; 5) difficulty in bilateral movements; and 6) difficulty in moving when a patient feels unpleasant[9]. As for the symptoms, patients are "having difficulty in moving without

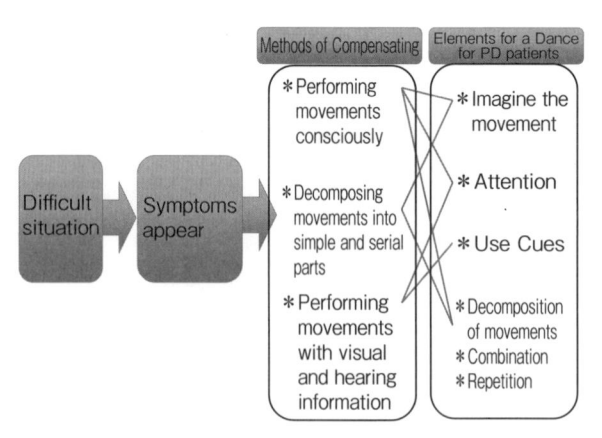

Figure 2 Elements for the PD Dance

visual cues," "cannot cope with an unexpected situation," "cannot do one thing while doing another thing," "freezing of gait," and "cannot keep good balance." As for the movements necessary to response to these characteristics, quick switching movements, combination movements, parallel movements, complex movements of the fingers, walking, and balancing were pointed out. Furthermore, by combining the methods such as "move consciously," "practicing decomposed movement into simple parts" and "appropriately using visual and auditory information" [9], as the method of compensating for symptoms of PD patients, with the characteristics of dance, the four elements and methods necessary for the Neurodance were formulated as follows:

1) Imagine the movement
　・Give verbal cues to the participants so that they can imagine some movements in daily activities.
2) Attention
　・Give them verbal cues so that they can be conscious about their movement.
　・Give them a clear cue immediately before the action.
3) Use cues
　・Determine the line of vision (Visual)
　・Move to the rhythm (Auditory)
　・Patting (Tactile)
4) Decomposing of movements and combination of movements, and repetition
　・Repeat the decomposed movement several times.
　・Repeat the combined movement several times.

In the next section, how these four elements should be incorporated into the session is explained based on the following dance structure.

Table Elements and Structure of the Neurodance

Composition	Variety	Part of Body	Movement	Element
Warming up	The Stretch and Relax Dance	Body trunk Upper limbs Lower limbs	Strech Rotation Flexibility Relaxation	Imagine the movement Attention
	The Patting Dance	Body trunk Upper limbs Lower limbs Neck	Patting Strech	Use cues (Tactile) Use cues (Visual) Attention
Main Exercise	The Heel and Toe Dance	Lower limbs	Strech Switching Combination	Imagine the movement Attention Use cues (Auditory) Decomposition Combination Repetition
	The Arm and Finger Dance	Upper limbs	Switching Combination Complex movements Both hands movements Parallel movements	Imagine the movement Attention Use cues (Auditory) Decomposition Combination Repetition
	The Hand towel Dance	Body trunk Upper limbs Lower limbs	Switching Combination Both hands movements Parallel movements Rotation	Imagine the movement Attention Use cues (Auditory) Use cues (Visual) Decomposition Combination Repetition
	The Balance Dance	Body trunk Upper limbs Lower limbs	Balance Switching Combination Both hands movements Parallel movements	Imagine the movement Attention Use cues (Auditory) Use cues (Visual) Use cues (Tactile) Decomposition Combination Repetition
	The Walking Dance	Upper limbs Lower limbs	Walking Balance Switching Combination Parallel movements	Imagine the movement Attention Use cues (Auditory) Combination Repetition
Cooling Down	The Swaying Dance	Body trunk Upper limbs Lower limbs	Relaxation Strech	Imagine the movement Attention

Structure of the Neurodance (Table)

The structure of the Neurodance consists of the three parts of warming up, main exercise, and cooling down. Because PD patients get tired easily, a period of 40–50 minutes is appropriate. At the main exercise, it is important to schedule break times (deep breathing, stretch, and relaxation). In order for PD patients to practice the dance with ease, it is important that the exercised areas of the body are not biased in relaxation, moving from periphery to central parts and form a sitting to a standing positions.

1) Warming up

PD patients tend to lack exercise due to the impairment of movement and this will cause stiffness of muscles and joints[10]; therefore, it is very important to warm the body and relax muscles and joints. Give them verbal cues to prompt the image of movement in order to make them move their bodies as much as possible. Imagining is good for exercise preparation and patients can be easily conscious of their movements by significantly moving their bodies[11]. The main feature of the Neurodance warm-up is patting[12]. Patting is for the purpose of stimulating the body and making PD patients confirm the outer appearance and size of their body before the movement of the development stage, and as a result, it helps them move more easily[8].

2) Main exercise

The main exercise consists of rapid switching movements, combination movements, complex movement of the fingers, movement of both hands, balancing, and walking, and it is mainly for the improvement of cognitive functions. This stage contains all elements necessary for the Neurodance structure because in this structure, the movements are broken down, and simpler movements are gradually combined, difficulty levels and rhythms are varied and PD patients are prompted to imagine the movement, although the Neurodance structure is difficult for them, they can perform it, repeating it without getting bored.

3) Cooling down

The cooling down stage is to relax and rest the body. To be conscious of and feel one's own body is the most important in relaxation. For that purpose, it is necessary to meditate with words evoking pleasant images.

Conclusion

We believe that the Neurodance system comprehensively contains the elements necessary for PD rehabilitation. Even if they cannot perfectly perform all the movements, they can easily participate in the session and pleasantly experience all contents only by moving the body to music. The purpose of this rehabilitation program is for the PD patients to easily, happily and continuously participate. The next task is to verify the effects of the Neurodance system on daily living activities from the viewpoints of various physical functions.

(Hiroko Hashimoto)

References

1) Japanese Society of Neurology (ed) : Parkinson-Byou Tiryou Guideline 2011 [Treatment Guideline for Parkinson's Disease 2011]. Igaku-Shoin, 2011 (in Japanese)
2) Schrag A, et al : What contributes to quality of life in patients with Parkinson's disease? *J Neurol Neurosurg Psychiatry* 69 : 308-312, 2000
3) Westheimer O : Why dance for Parkinson's disease. *Top Geriatr Rehabil* 24 : 127-140, 2008
4) Hackney ME, et al : Effects of tango on functional mobility in Parkinson's disease—a preliminary study. *J Neurol Phys Ther* 31 : 173-179, 2007
5) Cooper JA, et al : Cognitive impairment in early, untreated Parkinson's disease and its relationship to motor disability. *Brain* 114 : 2095-2122, 1991
6) Shiotsuki H : Parkinson-Byou ni tsuite (Genin/Tiryou/Byoutai) [Parkinson's Disease Outlook (Cause/Treatment/Pathology]. *MB Med Reha* 135 : 1-9, 2011 (in Japanese)
7) Morris ME : Movement disorders in people with Parkinson disease—a model for physical therapy. *Phys Ther* 80 : 578-597, 2000
8) Yoshii H : Parkinson-Byou no Ninchikinou Shougai ni taisuru Rehabilitation [Rehabilitation for Cognitive Function Disorder in Parkinson's Disease]. Yamamoto M : Parkinson-Byou [Parkinson's Disease]. Chugai-Igakusha, pp283-294, 2003 (in Japanese)
9) Takabatake S, Tomatsu Y, Naito Y, et al : Parkinson-Byou Toujisha ni okeru Nichijyou Seikatsu no Konnan to Sono Tokusei [Difficulties in activities of daily living of patients with Parkinson's disease and its characteristics]. *Jpn J Osaka Occup Ther Assoc* 23 : 57-63, 2009 (in Japanese)
10) Nagaoka M : Parkinson-Byou no Rehabilitation [Rehabilitation in Parkinson's Disease]. *MB Med Reha* 135 : 11-18, 2011 (in Japanese)
11) Sakamoto C, et al. : Lee Silverman Ryouhou (LSVT BIG) niyoru Parkinson-Byou no Rehabilitation [Rehabilitation for Patients with Parkinson's Disease with Lee Silverman Therapy (LSVT BIG)]. *MB Med Reha* 135 : 61-65, 2011 (in Japanese)
12) Keus SHJ, et al : Evidence-based analysis of physical therapy in Parkinson's disease with recommendations for practice and research. *Mov Disord* 22 : 451-460, 2007

2 The Effectiveness of Dance for the People with Parkinson's Disease

Introduction

Hackney and Earhart[1] at University of Washington reported that the balance ability of the Parkinson's disease (PD) patients who participated 20 times in the class of the tango, as compared with the PD group that only focused on the physical exercise, was improved and their score of Unified Parkinson's disease rating scale (UPDRS), and Timed Up and Go test (TUG) were higher. TUG is used for the evaluation of the risk of falling by measuring the time to walk three meters and return.

Recently, the effects of dance to improve the motor function and balance ability of PD patients have been noted. **Table** is a summary of the study on the effects of dance for PD patients in recent years. Difference of effect has been reported by the presence or absence of partners and types of dance such as the waltz and tango. These reports show that the effects of dance were relatively long lasting and improved quality of life (QOL) in many PD patients.

As a total assessment index of function of patients with PD, UPDRS has been widely used internationally. However, since UPDRS takes time for the evaluation, it was necessary to study to determine the effect of short-term before and after that was carried out in a group using dance. Therefore, the Neurodance study group has decided to implement by combining the evaluations that include the three factors, and they are as follows: 1) the total time of the evaluation of one person that can be carried out in about 30 minutes, 2) a significant correlation with the UPDRS is found, 3) measuring the motor imagery. The motor imagery ability assessment has been used in the field of rehabilitation for PD infrequently. However, as in our initial investigation, whether motor imagery can be used as an indicator of the effect of dance, has shown that the use of image capacity, in its role in rehearsal of action and behavior is an effective measurement.

Based on the above point of view, we performed Timed Motor test (TMT) and TUG as a motor function assessment, Functional Reach test (FRT) as balance ability assessment, and Mental Rotation task (MRT) of hand as an image capability assessment.

In addition, we have conducted a facial expression recognition task and examined the prefrontal cortex activity, due to differences in the way of dance appreciation. MRT of hand and facial expression recognition task are unique evaluation developed origi-

Table Summary of the Study on the Effects

	Title	Journal	Year	Subjects	Methods and Results
Hackney, et al.	Effects of tango on functional mobility in Parkinson's disease : a preliminary study	J Neurol Phys Ther	2007	19 PD patients	Comparing the effects of physical exercise group and tango dance group. Twenty times trials. UPDRS improved significantly in both groups. BBS improvement found only group of tango, TUG was also seen improvement trend.
Hackney, et al.	Short duration, intensive tango dancing for Parkinson disease : an uncontrolled pilot study	Complement Ther Med	2009	14 PD patients	Conducted ten times over two weeks of tango once 90 minutes. Main Outcome Measures included BBS, UPDRS, gait velocity, functional ambulation profile, step length, stance and single support percent of gait, TUG, and 6MWT. As the results of evaluation, BBS and UPDRS were improved, and extension of stride during walking was observed.
Marchant, et al.	Effects of a short duration, high dose contact improvisation dance workshop on Parkinson disease : A pilot study	Complement Ther Med	2010	11 PD patients	Performed for ten times over a period of two weeks of dance once 90 minutes led by a dancer. Evaluated UPDRS III, TUG, BBS, STS, and Walking Improvement was shown on balance and motor function items of the UPDRS.
Hackney, et al.	Effects of dance on movement control in Parkinson's disease : A comparison of Argentine tango and American ballroom	J Rehabil Med	2010	58 moderate PD patients	Randomly divided into two groups to participate in the waltz and the tango, twice a week, carried out over 13 weeks 20 dance lessons of one hour. Evaluation included, UPDRS, BBS, TUG, and 6MWT. Compared to the control group in both groups, a large improvement was shown on the 6MWT and BBS. The tango group improved as much or more than those in the waltz group on several measures.

Table cont.

	Title	Journal	Year	Subjects	Methods and Results
Hackney, et al.	Effects of dance on balance and gait in severe Parkinson disease : a case study	Disabil Rehabil	2010	one male severe PD patient, 86-year-old, Hoehn-Yahr Stage IV	Implementation of 20 lessons over a period of ten weeks tango dance with a partner of one hour once. Evaluation included, UPDRS, BBS, 6MWT, FRT, PDQ39, and ZBI. As the evaluation results, BBS, and 6MWT, FRT were improved. Increased the confidence of balance and improved the quality of life were reported as measured by the PDQ39. As other, caregivers hope to continue to dance, but worried about increase the care burden.
Heiberger, et al.	Impact of a weekly dance class on the functional mobility and on the quality of life of individuals with Parkinson's disease	Front Aging Neurosci	2011	11 severe PD patients	Verification of the immediate effects of dance, and the effects of long-term after the 8-month implementation of the dance once a week with a professional dancer. Evaluated UPDRS III, TUG, SeTa, and the QOLS. Total score of the UPDRS was improved. QOLS shown positive result.
Hackney, et al.	Effects of dance on gait and balance in Parkinson's disease : a comparison of partnered and non partnered dance movement	Neurorehabil Neural Repair	2011	39 mild-moderate PD patients	Verification of the effects of the difference in the case of dance alone and dance with a partner on tango dance. Twice a week, conducted over ten weeks and 20 lessons of one hour dance once. Evaluated UPDRS, BBS, TUG, 6MWT, TS, and OLS. Stride speed, BBS and walking were improved in both groups; however, people who danced with partners expressed more enjoyment and intention of continuation.

UPDRS : Unified Parkinson's disease rating scale, TUG : Timed Up and Go test, BBS : Berg Balance scale, STS : Sit-to-Stand test, SeTa : Semitandem test, QOLS : Quality of Life scale, 6MWT : Six minute walk test, TS : Tandem stance, OLS : One Leg Stance, FRT : Functional Reach test, PDQ39 : Parkinson's disease questionnaire-39 items, ZBI : Zarit Burden Interview

nally by the authors of this book.

The Effectiveness of the Neurodance for People with Parkinson's Disease

We compared the results of each evaluation of before and after the Neurodance. Subjects and methods are as follows:

1) Subjects
Subjects are twelve PD patients (3 males and 9 females). The mean age was 64.56 ± 7.00 years.

2) Methods
In the regular meeting of PD patient's association at Hiroshima prefecture branch, the Neurodance was performed for about 40 minutes by instructors with experience of teaching dance for many years.

We recorded and compared body functions and changes in cognitive function on before and after the Neurodance.

1. Motor function

1) Timed Motor test (TMT)
TMT consists of (a) walking, (b) writing, (c) single and double-handed pegboard performance, (d) finger tapping, and (e) rapid alternating forearm movements. Haaxma et al[2] reported that TMT is equally effective as well as UPDRS-III, but requiring less time than the scale. In this study, the finger tapping task and pegboard task are used as an evaluation of TMT. As a result of the verification, there were no significant difference between before and after dance of each evaluation.

2) Timed Up and Go test (TUG)
TUG is a test to assess the performance of general physical function such as mobility, balance, and locomotor performance in elderly people with balance disturbances. More specifically, it assesses the ability to perform sequential motor tasks relative to walking and turning. The individual must stand up from a chair, walk a distance of three meters, turn around, walk back to the chair and sit down—all performed as quickly and as safely as possible.

As a result of the verification, a significant difference was observed in the TUG operation time, after dance was implemented (**Figure 1** top). In our developing Neurodance, because the proportion patients need to be in the sitting position was higher using, the focus was on upper extremity, with a prediction in the improvement of motor function in that assessment. However, no changed was shown in upper extremity improvement, yet in overall result on improve effect was observed in the general physical function related to walking ability.

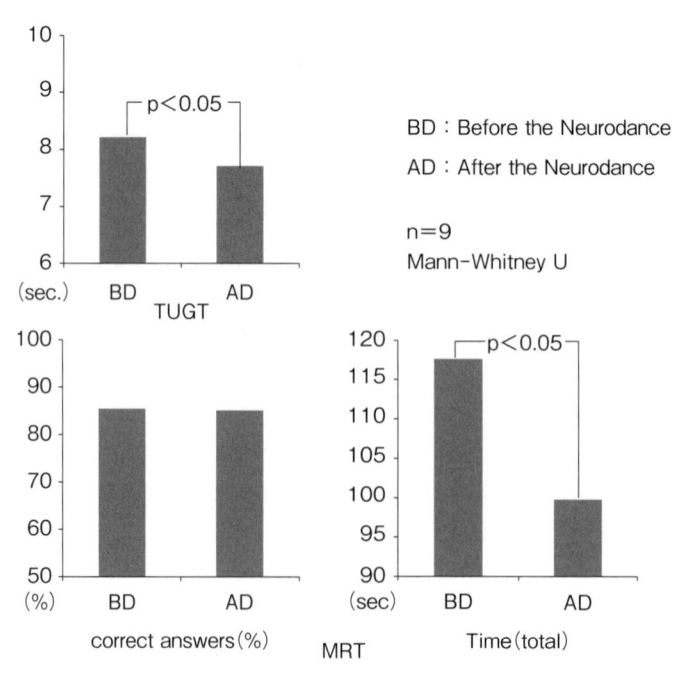

Figure 1 Comparison of Before and After the Dance on TUG and MRT

In previous studies, the effect of dance for PD patients on BBS (Berg Balance Scale) have been reported multiple (table). By considering BBS is consists of the sub-items such as picking something up from the floor, the rotating, tandem standing position, it will be conceived that the Neurodance is effective in improving the complex motor function.

2. Balance ability

FRT (Functional Reach test)

The Functional Reach test is a quick screen for determining risk of falls in elder people and neuromuscular disease patients. The patient is instructed to stand next to, but not touching the wall and to position the arm that is closer to the wall at 90° of shoulder flexion with a closed fist. Place the ruler horizontally on the wall and secure appropriately. Record the starting position at the 3rd metacarpal head on the ruler. And ask the patient to reach forward as far as he can without taking a step and keeping his hands in a fist shape. The location of the 3rd metacarpal is marked and recorded. As a result of the verification, there was no significant difference before and after the dance.

3. Motor Imagery

MRT (Mental Rotation task) of hand

The Mental Rotation task of hand is unique method of using visualization prior to movement, developed by the authors, originally with reference to the study of Helimich et al.[3] It is used for measuring the time until the answer by subject pressing the keyboard, hand presented on the computer screen whether left or right.

The task is made up of 48 photographs. Using the photographs of the left hand and the right hand which was rotated 360 degrees in 45-degree increments, dorsum of the hand, from the thumb side. After the hand picture was displayed on the screen of the personal computer, reaction time is measured (msec) until pressing the button.

Comparing before and after the dance, after dance, correct answers score (%) had significantly increased and time (total sec) had significantly shortened (**Figure 1** bottom).

It is well-known that during mental rotation performance premotor cortex, supplementary motor area are activated, these areas are involved in preparation and planning of movement. In this dance, it is possible that the time of the MRT of the hand was shortened by the performer while the operation instructor encouraging the subject to predict what to do next.

4. Recognition of facial expression

When you have positive impression on the facial expression of others, the opportunity to talk may increase. Conversely, you do not want to talk when you perceive angry face of others. Using computer morphing technology, we have investigated the changes in facial expression recognition of others before and after dancing[4].

First of all, using computer morphing animation creation software "Sqirlz Morph" (Xiberpix Inc.), we have created an ambiguous expression by combining expressions of joy, anger, and grief of people. In this task, the subject is presented in random order photographs of various mixing ratio of emotional facial expression, and subjects respond the impression for each expression by the semantic differential (SD) method.

The randomly arranged twenty pieces facial expression photographs which were morphed in the ratio of various ways, and presented every three seconds. After emotions aroused by the dance, we examined facial expression of others whether to look more positive in comparison with before dancing.

Comparing before and after the dance, anger score has significantly changed in four of eight of the PD patients after dance (**Figure 2** right). In addition, in the joy and grief score, the joy score has significantly changed in three of the eight PD patients (**Figure 2** left). As a result of this study, conclusions are that, when physical activity was increased by dance in using happy/angry, the expression of anger was more easily perceived. On the other hand, they feel joy rather than grief in using joy/sadness, recognizing of joy is more easily perceived.

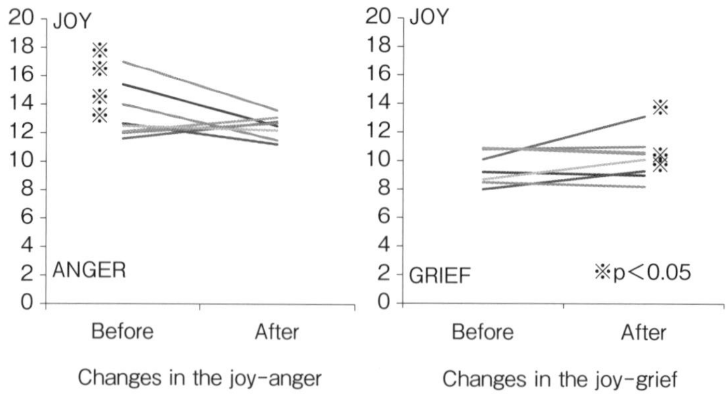

Figure 2　Changes in the Recognition of Facial Expressions in the Comparison Before and After, Doing Neurodance

5. Activity of the prefrontal cortex due to differences in the way of watching dance

Using near-infrared spectroscopy (NIRS), we examined the activity of the prefrontal cortex due to differences in the way of watching dance. The method is as follows;

1) Subjects

Subject is a PD patient (female), Septuagenarian. Disease duration was 28 years.
　Hoehn & Yahr stage: III, UPDRS 40.

2) Methods

For measurement, optical encephalography (Spectratech OEG-16 Spectratech Inc.), personal computer, and task presentation monitor were used. In a quiet place where it is easy to concentrate, the subject sits in a chair. Attached is the brain function measuring device to the forehead. We have each three sets of ninety seconds, with twenty seconds of watching video for each of the three conditions with a ten-seconds rest period between video viewing. Each condition consists of three sets of repeated three times of task and rest. The cerebral blood flow were recorded during each three conditions and compared by averaging.

　　Condition 1: Only watching the DVD video of the Neurodance.
　　Condition 2: Watching the DVD video with the aim to learn the Neurodance.
　　Condition 3: Watching the video of the natural landscape (scene of the sea) that is not related to dance.

　Figure 3 illustrates the average value for each condition. It can be seen that the high activity in condition 2, which has been watched with the focus to learn the Neurodance. In recent studies have shown that the left prefrontal cortex is involved in the prediction of future rewards[5].

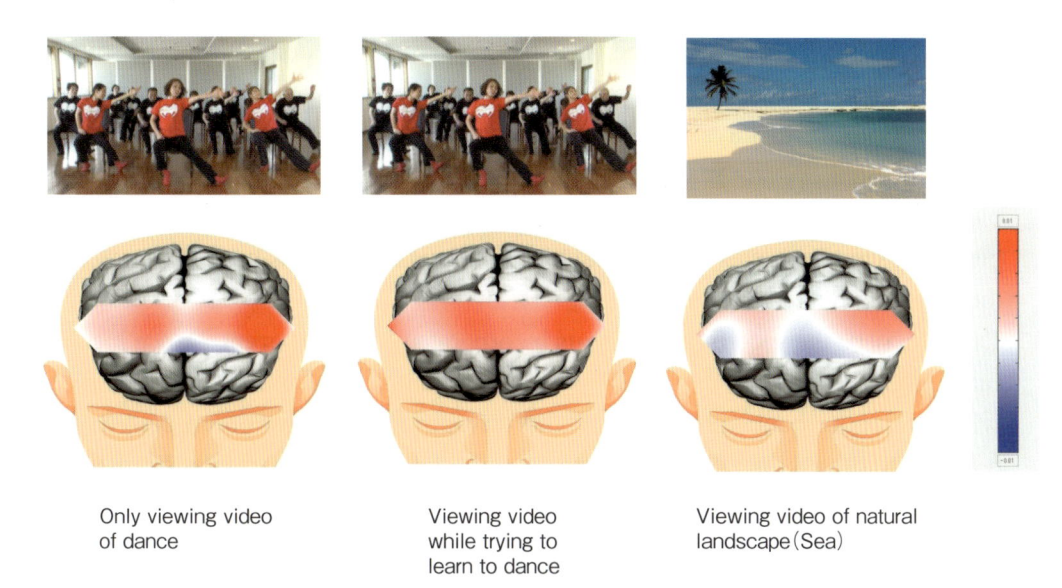

| Only viewing video of dance | Viewing video while trying to learn to dance | Viewing video of natural landscape (Sea) |

Figure 3　Activity in the Prefrontal Cortex during Viewing video (PD patient)

This subject has experienced the Neurodance, and was vocally indicated that it was a lot of fun. There may be a possibility this patient has previous experience of dance; therefore, by dance experience the left prefrontal cortex was activated. It would also be considered that left prefrontal cortex area, relates to the language area when subject is trying to remember the dance.

Why the Neurodance is Effective in PD Patients?

As a result of the verification, significant improvement of motor function of the upper limbs was not observed immediately after performing the Neurodance. However, significant change was observed in the score of TUG and MRT of hand associated with the hand imagery. In these changes, the reaction time became faster in all the tasks.

It can be considered that one of the reason why the reaction time has become faster, is that of involvement of the frontal lobe function being related to the motor imagery.

Earhart[6] has pointed out the possibility of the following five factors about why there were effects of dance in PD patients in the effect validation study with a focus on dance tango.

1) The practice of dance may facilitate activation of areas that normally show reduced activation in PD. Healthy controls who learned to dance tango showed a shift in cortical activation, with increased activity in the premotor and supplementary motor areas during imagined walking following a series of tango lessons[7]. There are cues to increase the attention by dance.
2) In addition to attentional cues, people with PD can utilize other forms of cueing to

improve movement performance. These cues may be auditory, visual, or somatosensory[8]. Such cues have been postulated to bypass the diseased basal ganglia and utilize alternate pathways[9,10].

Rhythmic auditory stimulation is known to enhance walking performance in people with PD[11-14]. Auditory cues may bypass the basal ganglia and access the supplementary motor area via the thalamus[15] or they may access premotor cortex via the cerebellum[16].

3) Dance may be the specific movements incorporated in the program. Dance incorporates practice of many functional movements that people with PD may struggle with, including backward walking and turning. Dance may be an activity that requires multitasking. People with PD are known to have particularly difficulty walking while performing a secondary task[17-21], but practice in multitasking situations can improve performance[22,23]. In addition, the leader must be continually planning ahead to execute the next step in the sequence, while the follower must wait for and interpret signals from the leader regarding the next step.

4) The cardiovascular effects of dancing tango have also been proved, and tango elevates heart rate to approximately 70% of maximum which is in the appropriate range for aerobic training[24].

5) Dance may enhance social support networks, thereby contributing to improve QOL. The social nature of dance may also be important for promoting long-term participation in those with PD. Dance not only expands older individuals' repertoire of physical activity, but may also foster further community involvement, personal development, and self-expression[25].

As introduced in this report, studies on the effects of dance for PD patients show very compelling results. In the near future, as the relationship of dance with emotional function and frontal lobe function becomes more clear, in which the authors are putting emphasis on, further effective rehabilitation that combines with medicine would be provided.

(Hideki Miyaguchi, Shinichi Takabatake)

References

1) Hackney ME, et al : Effects of tango on functional mobility in Parkinson's disease: a preliminary study. *J Neurol Phys Ther* 31 : 173-179, 2007
2) Haaxma CA, et al : Comparison of a timed motor test battery to the Unified Parkinson's Disease Rating Scale-III in Parkinson's disease. *Mov Disord* 23 : 1707-1717, 2008
3) Halmich RC, et al : Cerebral compensation during motor imagery in Parkinson's disease. *Neuropsychologia* 45 : 2201-2215, 2007
4) Konishi A : Waraikatudou ga Tasha no Hyojyo-ninchi ni Oyobosu Eikyo [Effects of laughter in cognition of others' facial expression]. Graduate thesis of Hiroshima University 16 : 7-12, 2011
5) Ueda K, et al : Brain activity during expectancy of emotional stimuli: an fMRI study.

Neuroreport 14：51-55, 2003
6) Earhart GM：Dance as therapy for individuals with Parkinson disease. *Eur J Phys Rehabil Med* 45：231-238, 2009
7) Sacco K, et al：Motor imagery of walking following training in locomotor attention. The effect of 'the tango lesson.' *NeuroImage* 32：1441-1449, 2006
8) Nieuwboer A, et al：Cueing training in the home improves gait-related mobility in Parkinson's disease：the RESCUE trial. *J Neurol Neurosurg Psychiatry* 78：134-140, 2007
9) Cunnington R, et al：Movement-related potentials in Parkinson's disease：presence and predictability of temporal and spatial cues. *Brain* 118：935-950, 1995
10) Debaere F, et al：Internal vs external generation of movements：differential neural pathways involved in bimanual coordination performed in the presence or absence of augmented visual feedback. *NeuroImage* 19：764-776, 2003
11) Thaut MH, et al：Rhythmic auditory stimulation in gait training for Parkinson's disease patients. *Mov Disord* 11：193-200, 1996
12) McIntosh GC, et al：Rhythmic auditory-motor facilitation of gait patterns in patients with Parkinson's disease. *J Neurol Neurosurg Psychiatry* 62：22-26, 1997
13) Rochester L, et al：The attentional cost of external rhythmical cues and their impact on gait in Parkinson's disease：effect of cue modality and task complexity. *J Neural Transm* 114：1243-1248, 2007
14) Baker K, et al：The effects of cues on gait variability—reducing the attentional cost of walking in people with Parkinson's disease. *Parkinsonism Relat Disord* 14：314-320, 2008
15) Nieuwboer A, et al：Is using a cue the clue to the treatment of freezing in Parkinson's disease? *Physiother Res Int* 2：125-134, 1997
16) Chuma T, et al：Motor learning of hands with auditory cue in patients with Parkinson's disease. *J Neural Transm* 113：175-185, 2006
17) Bloem BR, et al：The "posture second" strategy：A review of wrong priorities in Parkinson's disease. *J Neurol Sciences* 248：196-204, 2006
18) Galletly R, et al：Does the type of concurrent task affect preferred and cued gait in people with Parkinson's disease? *Aust J Physiother* 51：175-180, 2005
19) Canning CG：The effect of directing attention during walking under dual task conditions in Parkinson's disease. *Parkinsonism Relat Disord* 11：95-99, 2005
20) Rochester L, et al：Attending to the task：interference effects of functional tasks on walking in Parkinson's disease and the roles of cognition, depression, fatigue, and balance. *Arch Phys Med Rehabil* 85：1578-1585, 2004
21) O'Shea S, et al：Dual task interference during gait in people with Parkinson disease：effects of motor versus cognitive secondary tasks. *Phys Ther* 82：888-897, 2002
22) Silsupadol P, et al：Training of balance under single- and dual-task conditions in older adults with balance impairment. *Phys Ther* 86：269-281,2006
23) Wu T, et al：Neural correlates of dual task performance in patients with Parkinson's disease. *J Neurol Neurosurg Psychiatry* 79：760-766,2008
24) Peidro RM, et al：Tango：modificaciones cardiorrespiratorias durante el baile. *Rev Argent Cardiol* 70：358-363, 2002
25) Nadasen K："Life without line dancing and the other activities would be too dreadful to imagine"：an increase in social activity for older women. *J Women Aging* 20：329-342, 2008

3. Video DVD "Let's Enjoy PD Dance!" Description of the Contents and Points

This Video DVD is divided into nine sections.
"Let's Enjoy PD Dance!" (whole session, 35 minutes)
  1 : The Stretch and Relax Dance
  2 : The Patting Dance
  3 : The Heel and Toe Dance
  4 : The Arm and Finger Dance
  5 : The Hand towel Dance
  6 : The Balance Dance
  7 : The Walking Dance
  8 : The Swaying Dance

"Let's Enjoy PD Dance!" is a session of 35 minutes which consists of eight parts. This dance is made up of the movements necessary to improve movements of patients of Parkinson's disease (PD). These movements are supposed to be enjoyable for them.

Following 1-8 explain important points of each part. Explanation shows the points about the movement of the Video DVD and the purpose of each part of the dance.

【Basic Posture】

Basic posture is important in any part of dance.

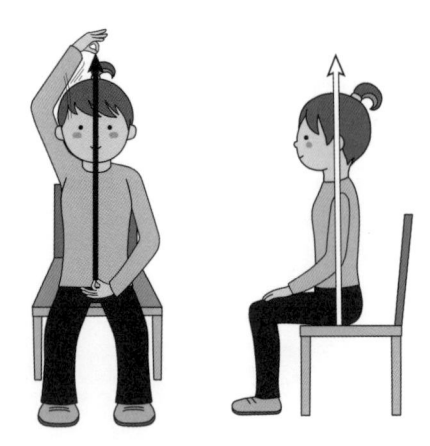

★Imagine the top of your head is being pulled by a string to the ceiling.
Sit down and straighten yourself up.

【1 : The Stretch and Relax Dance】

In this part, you will move your body greatly, and it will continue to increase the flexibility. This dance consists of the movements which warm your body, and stretch the muscles, such as stretching up and down or back and forth and bending or twisting the body to the right and left.

Draw a Big Eight

Pretend you are slowly drawing the character of a lateral 8 in the air with your both hands as large as possible!

★ Twist your body well.

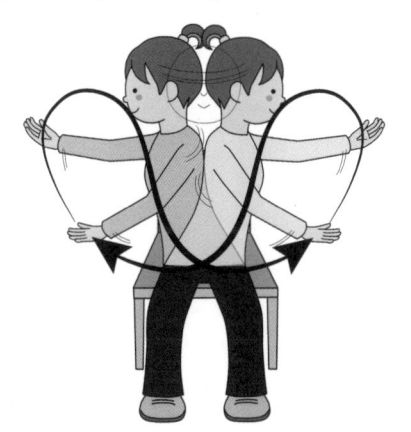

Push a Big Rock

Imagine yourself to push a large rock in front of you forward!

★ Use abs and back muscles.

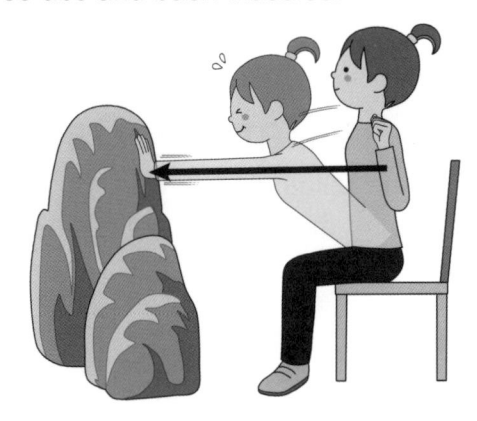

Like a Spring

Try to move as if you are a spring, make your body small and then stretch out!

★ Move as large as possible. It needs the balance ability.

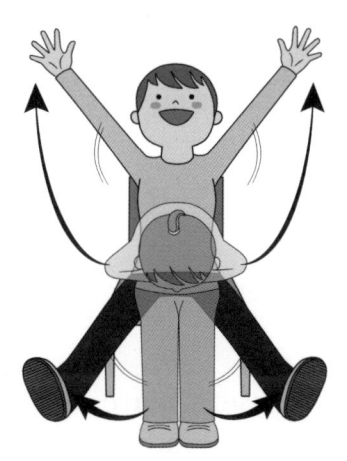

Throw a Balloon

Pretend you have a large balloon with your whole body!
★ Your back is rounded.

Toss the balloon high! Then look at the balloon.
★ Your back is extended. Use your dorsal muscles.

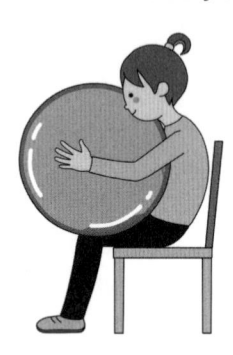

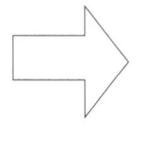

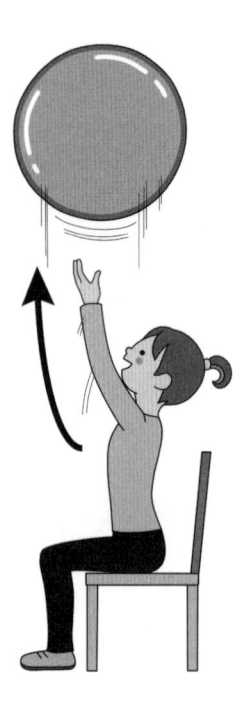

【2 : The Patting Dance】

This dance takes your power into your body and relaxes it, contracting and stretching of muscle, and patting each part of the body. The point is to "feel the body".

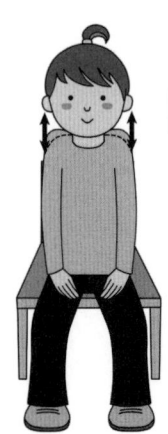

Up and Dawn

Raise your shoulders as if you shrugg your shoulders when it is cold.
Then drop your shoulders. It makes the shoulders relax.
★The movements relaxes muscles of your shoulders.

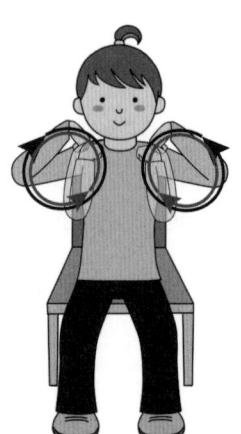

Circle, Circle, Circle!

Imagine yourself drawing circles with your elbows in the air. First draw big circles carefully and slowly.
Then draw small circles saying "circle, circle, circle!" It makes it easy to move.
★ The movements of the shoulders become smooth.

Patting Knees, Breasts, and Shoulders

Gradually, the switching of movement becomes faster.
Try to keep up with the rhythm.
★ It can be a brain exercise!

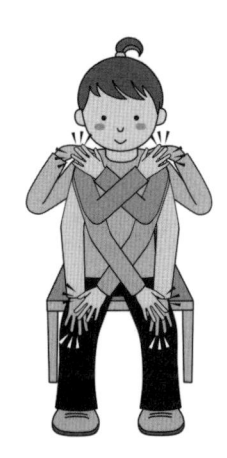

Neck Stretch

Slowly tilt your head to the right and left, and then turn your head to the right and left. Feel your muscles around your neck are stretched. Move slowly at your pace and do not overdo it.
★ It is a stretch of neck and shoulders.

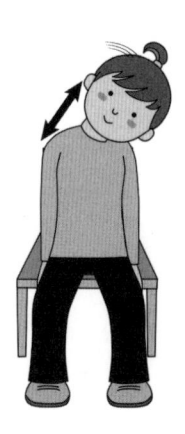

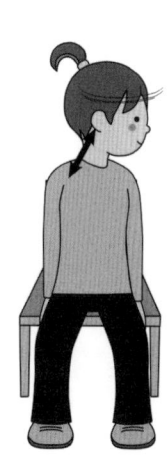

【3 : The Heel and Toe Dance】

This part of the dance is important exercise for muscles that is necessary for walking and keep your balance. This program consists of quick movements of the feet and coordinate movements of the feet foot and hands. Let's get into the rhythm.

Take Rhythm on Toe

Take rhythm on toe. First of all, get into the rhythm!
★ This is an exercise of tibialis anterior muscle.

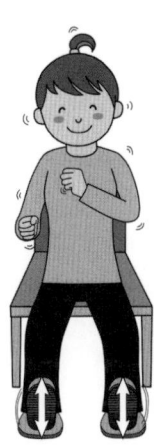

*Tibialis anterior muscle: The important muscle which raises a toe.

Pull the String of the Toe!

Put your heels down on the floor and raise toes as much as possible. Pretend as if your toes are being pulled by strings you hold.

★ This is an exercise of tibialis anterior muscle.

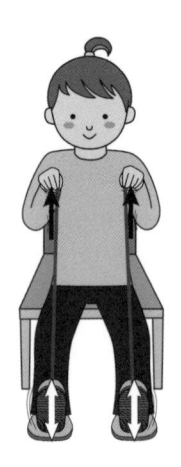

Open, Open tap-tap. Close, Close tap-tap

Pay attention to the movement of toe and heel. The fulcrum of the movement changes from the toe into heel.

★ This exercise includes complex movement of feet.

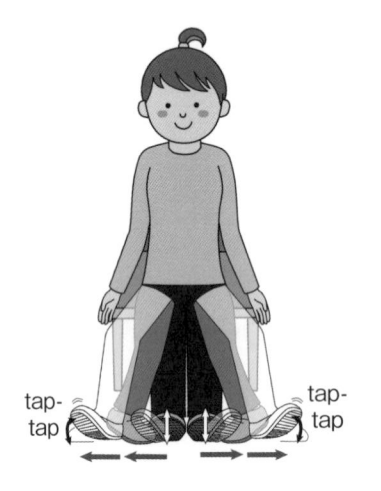

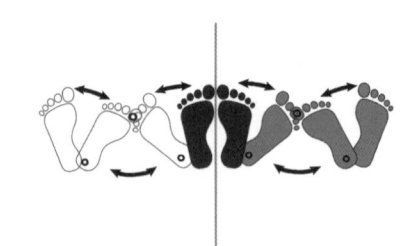

Let's Move Cool!

Put your heel down on the floor as far as possible, and then extend your knee.

Move your arms and legs as wide as possible.

★ With this exercise, your arms move while you are moving your legs (complex movements).

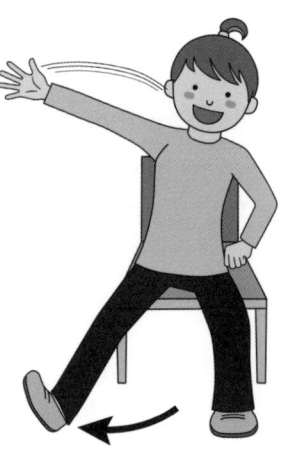

88   Part 3   Neurodance–Exercise for People with Parkinson's Disease

【4 : The Arm and Finger Dance】】

The aim of this dance is to learn complex movements and different movements in right- and left- limbs to rapidly respond to quick changes of movement. It works on cognitive function.

Rock and Paper

Clench your fingers firmly (like "the rock" of rock-paper-scissors), open your hands wide (like "the paper")! Put an accent on each movement and concentrate on switching of the movement.

★It makes you conscious of movement of the hands and that stimulates your brain.

Bending Finger

If you feel difficulty performing this exercise at first, practice slowly.

Do not give it up! The point of this exercise is to be able to bend your fingers one by one.

★ This is not merely the finger exercise, but the exercise of your brain.

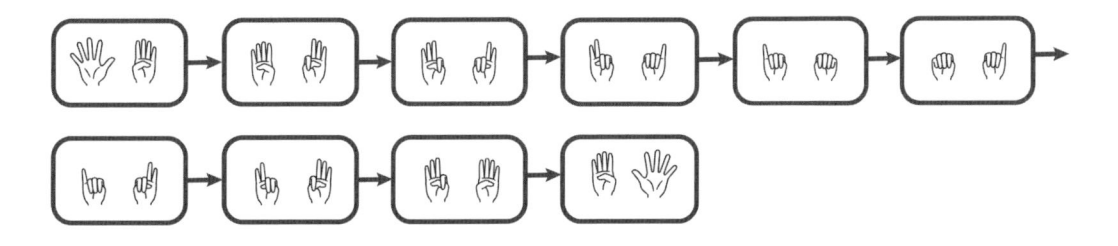

Two Beats, Three Beats

Be conscious of different movements in right and left arm. Challenge it the other way if you become to be able to do it.

★ This is an exercise of the brain.

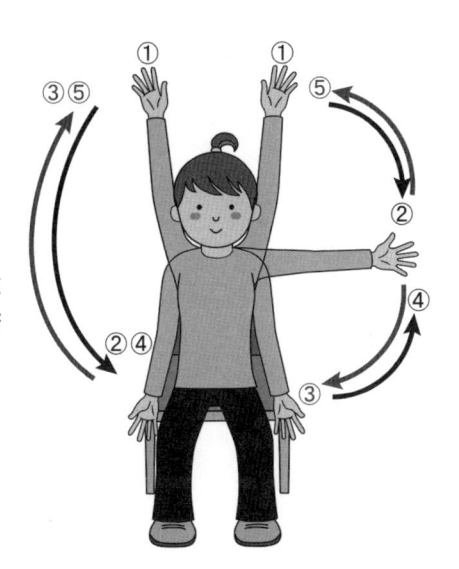

【5 : The Hand towel Dance】

In this part, you will twist your body and use your hands on the back with a hand towel. This exercise reduces the difficulties in movements which people with PD tend to have.

Using a hand towel facilitates your body movements because the towel plays the role of visual and tactile clues.

Pull your towel tight.

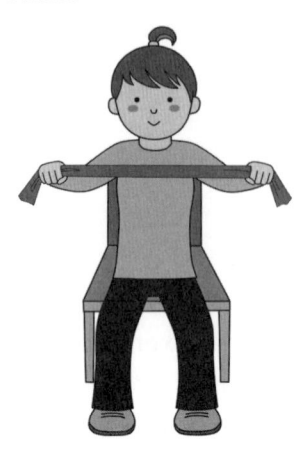

Look at the Back

Twist well your body as if you are showing your back to someone in front of you. Pull one side of the towel forward.

★ Twist your body well.

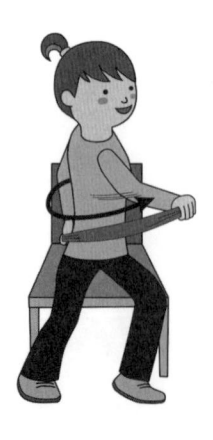

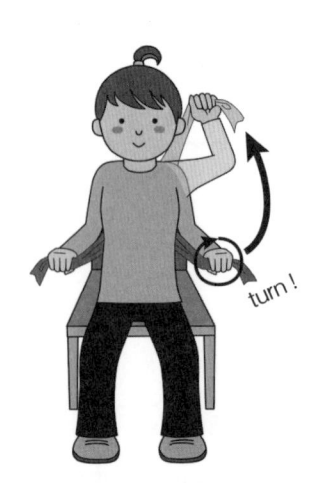

Have a Towel Diagonally on your Back

Turn your wrist. Be conscious of your body movement.

★ The point is the movement of the wrist.

Wash Your Back

Imagine yourself washing your back in the bath. Look at the point of the hand that you drew.

★Be conscious of the movement of the hand and the direction of the face.

Turn a Wrist Alternately

★The point is the movement of the wrist.

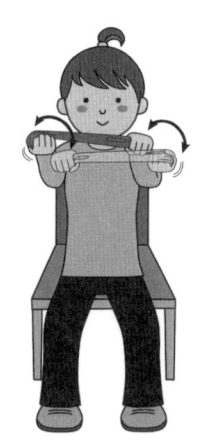

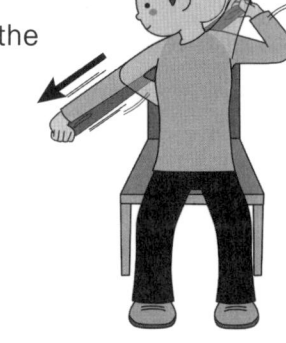

【Balance】

Knowing where the center of your body is helpful to keep your balance. Check the balance of the body while moving the center of gravity back and forth, right and left.

Basic Posture

Stand as if you raise your body from the navel.

Tighten the gluteus and relax the shoulders. Smile!! Excess power will fall out .

★ Be conscious of the center of the body.

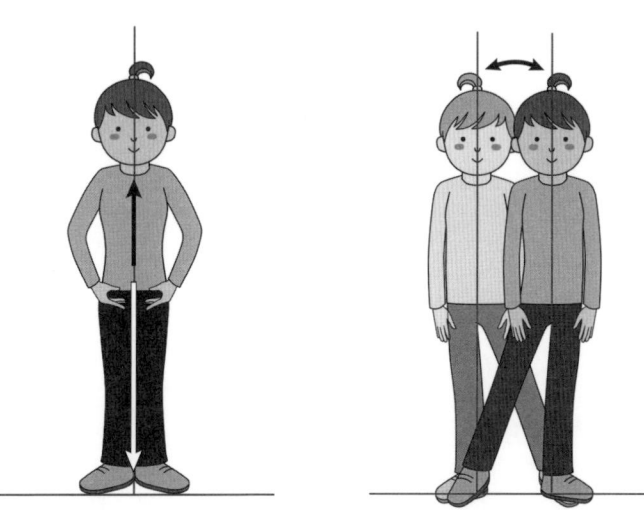

Check the balance of your body while moving the center of gravity.

Move the Center of Gravity (to the Right and left)

While moving your body to the right and left slowly, confirm your center of gravity.

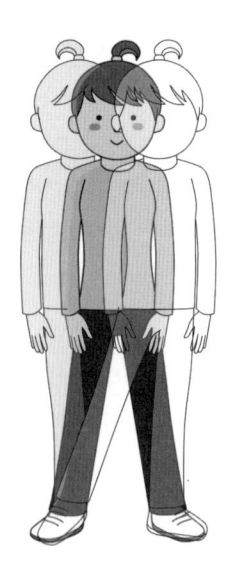

Toe Exercise

Strongly bend the toes.⇒Open it well slowly.⇒Grab a floor with the toes which are opened.
Regulate it so that the weight is equally on the sole.

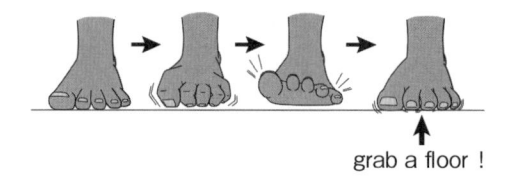

grab a floor !

Move the Center of Gravity (Forward and backward)

Open the toes well and apply the center of gravity forward a little while bracing the toe. Keep the heel resting on the floor. ⇒ Return to the basic posture.
★ Confirm your center of gravity of the body.

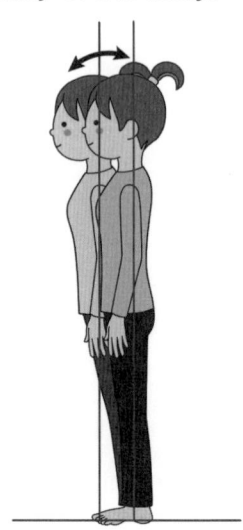

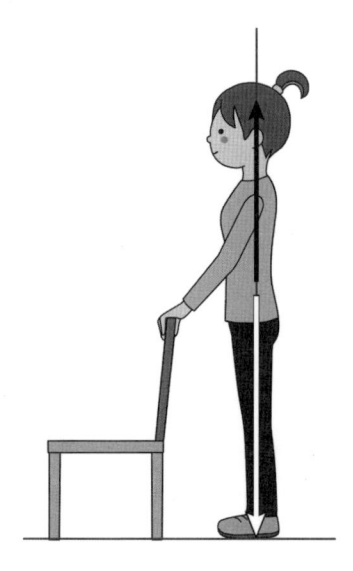

【6 : The Balance Dance】

This part develops the balance ability while seeking for the center of gravity of your body.

Imagine you are a ballet dancer!

Confirm first the posture while holding back of a chair as the support. If you get used to the exercise, you can do it without the support.

Forward, Right and Left, Backward (Tendu)

This movement is called "tendu" in ballet. Tendu means "stretched" or "pulled" in French.

Imagine someone is pulling your leg, and then put the leg forward, to the right and left, and backward.

★ Confirm the center of the body.

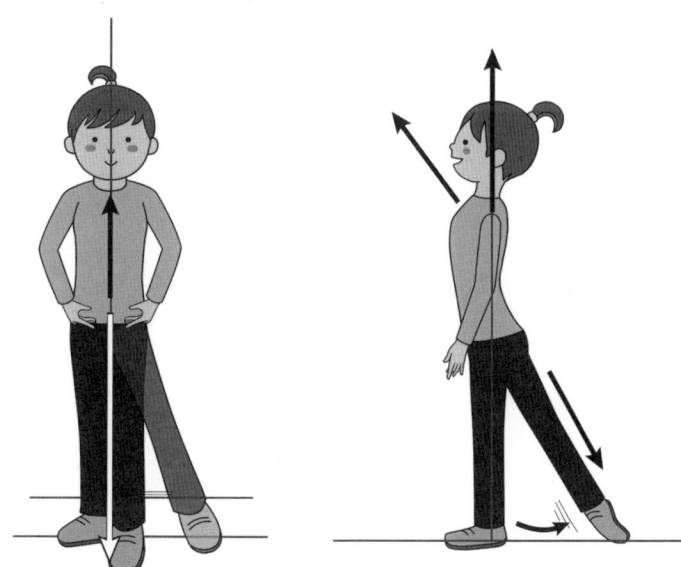

Flowers for you!

Move your center of gravity to the leg you have put forward, as if you give a flower to someone in front of you. Move your center of gravity to another leg as if you get a flower.

It is difficult to keep balance. Focus on your movements.

★ Confirm your center of gravity which moves forward and backward.

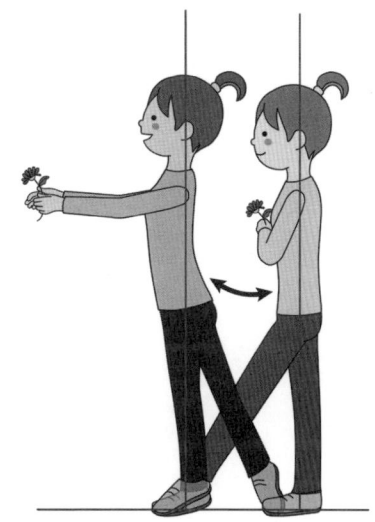

【7 : The Walking Dance】

This part makes it easy to walk in your everyday life.
Repeat it many times, moving the center of gravity forward and backward to the rhythm of the music.

Walk!!

Move your knees to the rhythm before walking. You can move your body up and down.
If you can follow the rhythm, swing your elbows. Then stamp your feet, you can do this while you are sitting on the chair.
★ Follow the rhythm!

Step Forward!!

Make sure your weight is on the foot you step with, and then to move your center of gravity backward. Center of gravity moves back and forth.
This movement is to prevent a fall and to make it easy to take the first step!

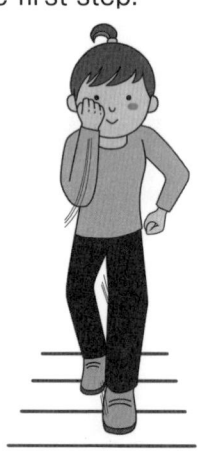

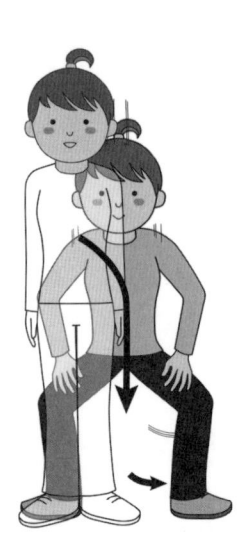

Step Right and Left!!

The center of gravity switches from the back and front to the right and left.
★Confirm the center of the body.

[8 : The Swaying Dance]

Imagine yourself floating in the sea like jellyfish or kelp, and sway your body. It is important to relax your body.

★There is no particular movement for this dance. Let's sway your body as you like.

■ How to use the Video DVD "Let's Enjoy PD Dance!"

You can change a combination of movements according to the state of your body and feelings. Try to dance all the parts when you have a lot of time. Try the "The Stretch and Relax Dance", "The Patting Dance", and "The Walking Dance" before going to shopping. Try the "The Heel and Toe Dance", and "The Arm and Finger Dance" as the brain exercise. You can make yourself a combination of dance.

Let's take the Neurodance-exercise in your life. Enjoy the dance, but do not over do it!

(Hiroko Hashimoto)

Choreographer : Hiroko Hashimoto
Instructors : Hiroko Hashimoto
　　　　　　　Naoko Shiromizu
　　　　　　　Aya Hashimoto
Performers : Kimiko Kajima, Machiko Shibata, Kiyoko Jyudai, Kayo Takeyasu,
　　　　　　　Yoshizo Takamatsu, Michiko Nakata, Hiroshi Nakanishi, Takehaya
　　　　　　　Hamana, Kazuko Yamada
Picture making : Somethingfun!
Special thanks to Koumyouike Studio Subaru

■ Video DVD for Neurodance-Exercise for People with Parkinson's Disease

This DVD disc is designed to play in either set-top DVD players or in DVD-ROM drives built into personal computers.

If the DVD does not play auto automatically, use your system's DVD player to open the program.

Neurodance-Exercise for People with Parkinson's Disease

発　　　行	2014年6月30日　第1版第1刷Ⓒ
編　　　集	高畑進一・宮口英樹
ダンス制作	橋本弘子
イラスト	めさきせいこ
発　行　者	青山　智
発　行　所	株式会社　三輪書店

〒113-0033　東京都文京区本郷 6-17-9　本郷綱ビル
☎ 03-3816-7796　FAX 03-3816-7756
http://www.miwapubl.com/

印　刷　所　　三報社印刷　株式会社

本書の内容の無断複写・複製・転載は，著作権の侵害となることがありますのでご注意ください．

ISBN 978-4-89590-478-0　C 3047

JCOPY ＜(社)出版者著作権管理機構　委託出版物＞
本書の無断複写は著作権法上での例外を除き禁じられています．複写される場合は，そのつど事前に，(社)出版者著作権管理機構（電話 03-3513-6969, FAX 03-3513-6979, e-mail: info@jcopy.or.jp）の許諾を得てください．